Men, Money,
and Medicine

MEN, MONEY, AND MEDICINE

by
Eli Ginzberg
with
Miriam Ostow

Columbia University Press
New York and London

Copyright © 1969 Columbia University Press

First printing 1969
Second printing 1971

ISBN 0-231-03366-4
Library of Congress Catalog Card Number: 79-101134
Printed in the United States of America

For
Carrie and
Moses Abramovitz

*A friend
loveth at all times*

Preface

The principal credit for turning primarily oral presentations to professional and lay audiences into written prose goes to Ruth Szold Ginzberg. To the extent that the volume has cohesion and is free of the informality of the spoken word, the merit is largely hers.

Miriam Ostow joined the staff in 1966 and has worked closely with me on most of the chapters. In addition, she revised and improved the entire manuscript. Her name on the title page indicates the nature of her contribution.

Two friends read the manuscript. Dr. Rashi Fein, Professor of Economics of Medicine, Harvard University, dispelled my doubts as to whether this interim effort should be published. Dr. Herbert E. Klarman, Professor of Public Health Administration, Johns Hopkins University, annotated the manuscript throughout and offered many other suggestions which added to the accuracy and readability of the book.

The primary source of the funding for the work underlying this book was the Manpower Administration, U.S. Department of Labor. Support was also received from the Planning Commission of the City of New York.

Eli Ginzberg, Director
Conservation of Human Resources

Columbia University
May, 1969

Contents

Men, Money,
and Medicine

~ I ~

Perspectives: A Retrospective View

The 1969 Report of the Council of Economic Advisors contains a small table which points up the important fact that in the twelve months between July 1, 1968 to June 30, 1969 the federal government spent a total sum of about $9.6 billion for Medicare and Medicaid for 19 million beneficiaries. In another section of the same Report, total expenditures for health and medicine in 1968 are calculated at $53 billion; recently Professor Herbert Klarman has suggested that these expenses approach $60 billion.

Even in a country with a gross national product of $871 billion, the expenditure of $60 billion for health services justifies interest, if not concern. While it may be true, as many people say, that nothing is more important than health, there are few objects of national spending on which the American public lavishes greater resources. In fact, only food, defense, and housing loom larger. Education, clothing, automobiles, and recreation all command less national effort and resources. The period since World War II has witnessed not only large and sustained increases in the absolute amounts spent for health services, but also a relative shift in combined consumer and governmental expenditures which has lifted the total from about 4.0 percent to 6.5 percent of GNP.[1]

These few facts and figures about post-World War II expenditures for health and medical services should go far to explain the burgeoning interest and concern of nonmedical groups, specialists, and laymen alike, in what is transpiring in the health field and what looms ahead. The Administrator of the Social Security System recently ventured the guess that hospital costs of $200 per patient day loom on the horizon. If such an eventuality is but a few years off, as he intimated, trends in medical care are a matter of national, not merely professional, concern.[2]

The essays that comprise this book represent views that were formulated after the passage of Medicare and Medicaid in 1965. But their roots go back a quarter of a century. This introductory chapter will seek to provide some perspective about the important postwar changes in the structure and functioning of health services. The viewpoint is that of an economist who has been concerned throughout the period with reconciling the aspirations of professional and political leaders to improve the quantity and quality of health services available to the American people within the context of our political system, which stresses freedom of choice of work, and the realities of our economic system, which places heavy reliance on competition in the market place.

The medical services of the Armed Forces in World War II provide a case illustration, albeit a limited one, of the strengths and weaknesses of a system of socialized medicine.

With money no object, with control over a significant proportion of the nation's medical manpower, with the triage of patients determined primarily by professional considerations, it was possible for the Armed Services to provide a high quality of medical care for the man in uniform and for some of his dependents. Many of the objectives of those who have sought to improve American medicine before and since were realized within the military system: strict control over the qualifications of physicians authorized to perform complicated procedures; the structuring of medical teams to optimize the talents and skills of the limited number of specialists; regionalization of hospitals so that patients could be treated close to their station and those who required more expert care could be transferred to major centers; the more effective integration of in-bed and ambulatory care to reduce the need for expanded hospital facilities.

Admittedly there were defects: physicians complained about having too little to do; some nurses complained that they were turned into administrators; patients complained that their hospital stay was unduly prolonged. The consultants discovered that some patients were diagnosed and treated too slowly, while others were overevaluated and overdoctored. But, on balance, the system must be judged successful. However, it had few lessons for peacetime since physicians and nurses are free to live and work where they prefer and patients cannot be ordered to seek medical attention from particular practitioners at specified facilities. A "rationalized" system of medical care requires control over both the purveyors of service and those who seek treatment.[3]

During the early postwar years President Truman threw his weight behind the Wagner-Murray-Dingell Bill, which sought to set up a national system of health insurance. A forerunner of this Bill was first advanced during the depressed 1930s when hospitals, together with the rest of the economy, were in serious financial plight, and its legislative proponents reintroduced it after the war. While credit for its defeat is usually given to the American Medical Association, which fought it tenaciously, a more reasonable interpretation is to look to the reform of hospital financing brought about by the rapid expansion of Blue Cross and commercial insurance. Prepaid hospital insurance went a long way to buttress the operating position of voluntary hospitals and Hill-Burton (passed in 1946) grants from the federal government and renewed philanthropic efforts provided much-needed funds for expansion and renovation.

The fact that the immediate postwar years (1945-50) saw substantial increases in per diem hospital costs, reflecting the prevailing inflation and the monetarization of hospital wages to make them more nearly competitive with other sectors of the economy, misled many to believe that the financial weakness of both the hospital and the consumer required drastic reform such as the enactment of compulsory health insurance. But, actually, when the hospitals brought their charges in line with their higher costs, their financial plight eased. And most, though not all, consumers found that they could pay their hospital bills through the insurance which they carried.[4]

This was the first of several instances on the health scene when a critical issue of an earlier day survived and continued to preoccupy the advocates of reform even after new institutions had come into being and had made the problem moot. But by December, 1951, when he created the Commission on the Health Needs of the Nation (Magnuson), President Truman recognized that alternative lines of progress had to be charted since national health insurance was dead—at least for the time being.[5]

A year before the appointment of the Magnuson Commission, at a symposium under the auspices of the American Economic Association on the "Economics of Medical Care," I warned about "the naive belief that alteration in the present methods of payment, even such a major change as the institution of compulsory government insurance, would contribute materially to the solution of the vast number of problems which are involved in raising the health standards of various sections of the country."[6]

No economist would minimize the importance of finances in expanding the quantity and quality of services that are available or in improving the access of persons with low incomes to these services. But it appeared necessary to remind this audience of economists that there were no tested standards to guide public action, because few planners distinguish clearly between "minimum," "adequate," and "desirable" services. Moreover, even while there clearly was a need for federal action, programs aimed at improving the standards of health of the American people had to be "adjusted to state and local conditions."[7]

The Magnuson Commission, which reported to the country just as General Eisenhower became President, set the second stage in the postwar panorama. Problems of restructuring the system of paying for medical care were muted, and in their place the role of the federal government in expanding the taut supply of physicians and other types of medical manpower and in expanding its support for medical research was highlighted. This became the new line.[8]

Several years previously the Committee on the Function of Nursing of Columbia University had stressed in its *Program for the Nursing Profession* that it was unwise to think of remedying existing and prospective shortages of nurses by expanding the conventional supply of registered nurses who earn their diploma after a course of three years. The real challenge, the Committee stated, was to change the structure of nursing services so that more persons with less extended training could be effectively utilized.[9]

A similar approach was used in an appraisal of the Magnuson Commission's emphasis on the need for a rapid expansion in physician manpower. "A judgment about the level of medical care is not the same as a judgment about the number of doctors, for the number of physicians is only one factor determining the level of medical care. New patterns of medical practice that will result in the improved utilization of the available supply of physicians provide a major opportunity for raising the level of medical care. . . . Moreover, no foreseeable increase in the number of graduates is likely by itself to solve some of the most serious types of shortages such as currently exist in rural areas and in many state hospitals."[10]

While the level of federal expenditures for medical research soon advanced to a level far beyond wildest expectations, the Magnuson Commission's recommendation that the federal government spend substantial sums on expanding the supply of physicians, nurses, and other health manpower was only modestly successful. It was not until 1963 that the government took significant steps in this direction, and even at the end of the 1960s it has not committed itself to support undergraduate medical or nurse education.

But to the surprise of many, over twoscore new medical schools have been opened in the interim or will soon open; nursing education, particularly at the baccalaureate and associate of arts levels, has likewise expanded significantly through state, local, and voluntary efforts. The expansion of allied health manpower has been on a scale that no one could have foreseen. This does not imply that as of 1969 the shortages, perceived or actual, have vanished. However, shortages which do not yield after two decades, despite a substantially increased supply of manpower, reflect, at least to the economist, a more complex phenomenon than the term "shortage" customarily connotes.

While financial concerns occupied the center of the stage in the early years after the war, and manpower stringencies the middle years, the last years have seen a preoccupation with the medical needs of the old and the poor. After many unsuccessful efforts, President Johnson succeeded in 1965 in winning congressional approval not only for Medicare but also for enlarging the role of the federal government in providing assistance to the states to pay for medical services for the poor through Medicaid. It is too late to raise again the objection leveled against the Magnuson Commission's report, that "it is never wise, and surely not in the case of the aged, to stress specific health services without reference to the ability of persons to meet their other essential needs."[11] And it is too early to know what lessons can be extracted from our emerging experience with this new legislation. But the cautionary note sounded in an early appraisal of the British Health Service appears to have merit: "We, too, must provide essential medical care for the poor, reduce the excessive medical costs for the middle class, and ensure the financial stability of our hospital system. But we must do more. We must continually strive for a higher quality of medical care and for improvements in preventive services. And we must seek to accomplish these purposes through an efficient and economical use of our resources. These are difficult objectives—and they cannot be accomplished by a single piece of legislation, not even by a host of legislative measures."[12]

The nub of this and many other issues in the realm of medical care is not whether more money, even more federal money, should be spent but "that there is no need to design grandiose plans and there is every reason to seek economical solutions for the specific problems that face us."[13] We have long confronted the need to improve medical care for older persons and for the poor, but one question has already been answered by the Congress. Medicaid is not an "economical solution." We hope that Medicare will prove viable.

From the vantage of economics a cautionary view was inevitable about the several panaceas that have been advanced during the last two decades to provide a high quality of medical care to all Americans—compulsory health insurance, governmental support for large-scale increases in the supply of medical manpower, or legislation focused specifically on meeting the needs of those who, because of age or ill fortune, do not have adequate resources of their own. Since even the affluent United States is characterized by scarce resources and since the distribution of income among individuals, groups, and communities is uneven, it has never been clear how large increases in governmental funding, large increases in medical manpower, or a combination of both would assure a satisfactory level of medical care for all. It would take more than money to attract physicians to areas of the country which they now avoid, and it would take many more millions than are now employed in the health services industry to provide a satisfactory level of care for all. The Magnuson Commission had, however, stated unequivocally: "We believe it is well within the economic potential of this country to provide itself with the finest system of medical care in the world, that the American people desire this and deserve no less." [14]

Underlying these views of the limited effectiveness of nostra and legislation to transform the system of medical care in the United States from one of mixed strengths and weaknesses to one in which poor and rich alike would have access to quality services at a reasonable cost is a recognition of the need of a demarcation between medical care and health—a demarcation that is not usually part of the thinking and planning of most medical reformers. An early formulation stated, "Health involves much more than the provision of adequate medical care, though medical care obviously has an important part to play in the establishment and in the maintenance of effective health.

It is an error, particularly for social scientists, to think of
health as an entity separate and distinct from the other
essential determinants of life—food, housing, education,
work."[15]

This position was elaborated in 1952 at the Centennial
Celebration of Mount Sinai Hospital in New York City in
a presentation on "Health, Medicine, and Economic Welfare." The following propositions were put forward at that
time.

> The marked improvement in the health of the popula-
> tion, measured in terms of greater longevity, lower mor-
> bidity, and greater effectiveness, largely reflects the rising
> standard of living which has characterized the United
> States . . . during the past many decades. . . . A diversified
> and enriched diet will probably contribute more to the
> health of the population of the South than any specific
> addition to medical resources, such as an increase in the
> number of doctors or the number of hospital beds.
>
> Only the experts have fully appreciated the extent to
> which most of the outstanding advances in health have
> been the by-products of basic research in bacteriology,
> chemistry, physics, and the other sciences rather than the
> results of clinical observation and experimentation.
>
> A sound attitude which permeates so much of the pub-
> lic's thinking about the right of every individual to essen-
> tial medical care derives from the conviction that all
> illness is an act of God . . . yet it is difficult to ignore com-
> pletely the issue of personal responsibility. . . . There are
> those who play hard and are willing to take large risks. . . .
> Good medical care can be provided only to those who
> have the desire and the intelligence—not to mention the
> means—to seek it. . . .
>
> The expansion of medical care is not the certain answer
> to better health. . . . Many challenges . . . lie in the area
> in which the purely medical becomes intertwined with the

economic and the social, as in the case of the need of the handicapped for jobs, the need of the chronically ill for homes, and the need of the mentally ill for a protective environment.

If maximum benefit for minimum cost is established as a criterion there are certainly serious deficiencies in the present organization of medical services. . . . [But] one must guard against overoptimism from structural changes. Medical care is expensive and will remain expensive. The only real control over costs is to keep the amount of medical services within bounds; to be sure that essential needs are met but that medical services do not expand beyond.[16]

From the early 1950s until the early 1960s, my colleagues and I explored various dimensions of human resources and manpower with only passing concern with medical problems. However, our explorations, particularly our large-scale investigation of *The Ineffective Soldier: Lessons for Management and the Nation,* reinforced our belief that "one cannot talk about effective therapy or care except in terms of the individual's capacity to function."[17]

A four-year term (1959-63) as a member of the national Mental Health Advisory Council, during which expenditures of the Institute of Mental Health grew from approximately $50 million to $180 million, gave me new perspectives on federal financing for research, demonstration, and training. It was early clear that the steady and rapid increases in expenditures for the National Institutes of Health would soon be reconsidered by a less-responsive Congress; this in fact occurred by the mid 1960s. It was also clear that it was easier to allocate rapidly rising congressional appropriations among competing claimants than to find research personnel with a record of accomplishment or with high potential. Moreover, questions arose about the system of project grants which made large sums available for specialized research while the financing of the basic biological sciences and medical education continued to be largely neglected.

In 1960, the Conservation staff responded to a request of the Federation of Jewish Philanthropies in New York City to review their affiliated hospitals and health agencies and to help the trustees chart directions for the future. The results of the study, published under the title *Planning for Better Hospital Care*,[18] called attention to the following major developments that loomed on the horizon: the diminishing role of philanthropy in the operating budgets of voluntary hospitals and the consequent onus on insurance and government to pay full costs; the certain rapid rise in hospital costs, estimated at 50 percent within the next five years; the need for medical school affiliation for hospitals that desire to remain in the vanguard; and the desirability of consolidations and mergers among neighboring hospitals to strengthen their capabilities and to avoid wasteful duplication. With more good luck than usually attends such studies, the principal recommendations aimed at consolidation were eventually put into effect in each of the three boroughs of the city. One unexpected development occurred: the trustees of Mount Sinai Hospital, impressed with the need for a medical school affiliation and balked at making one, decided to build their own medical school to assure the continued viability and vitality of this distinguished hospital. The new school opened in 1968.

This brief recapitulation indicates that the Conservation Project had had a continuing if uneven involvement in research in matters of health and medicine for over two decades when the Congress undertook new social legislation with the passage of Medicare and Medicaid in 1965. The new legislation left little question that, with much new money about to flow into the medical care system, the manpower stringencies that had characterized the system for many years would worsen, at least for a time. Involved as we were in manpower investigations and with our long-time interest and concern with the economics of health and medicine, it was inevitable that our research program be adjusted to enable us to reenter the medical arena. The recent publication of Greenfield and Brown, *Allied Health Manpower: Trends and Prospects,* is a first delivery.[19] The forthcoming volume on *Urban Health Services: The Case of New York* is a second installment.

The present effort is the first stage of a more systematic appraisal in *depth* of what we have learned from our more than a quarter-century of studies into the political economy of health.[20] All of the chapters were taken from presentations made after 1965 and consequently are responsive to present and emerging problems and trends. Each seeks to appraise recent efforts to improve our imperfect system of health care from our vantage of having studied similar and other efforts in the past and our understanding of the underlying directions of our pluralistic society and economy. The fact that much of what is said has a skeptical, sometimes critical, ring is not accidental. In each generation reformers shape their proposals and recommendations with little regard to the past. While the past is a poor guide for the future, planning that is uninformed by the past will repeat errors that might have been avoided. It is not heroic to look critically at contemporary proposals for medical reform but, as Keynes wrote years ago, if economists can be as useful as dentists, they have a worthwhile service to perform.

The several pieces that comprise this book are divided into four sections. In Part One, two themes predominate: What are reasonable expectations of a system of medical care for an affluent country which still confronts many unmet needs? And what have been some of the important financial and manpower transformations of the system as the nation has attempted to improve both the provision and distribution of health services?

In Part Two, the focus is on the critical role of the physician, male or female, who stands at the apex of the system and whose cooperation is required to accomplish significant changes. Particular attention is directed to the fact that physicians, like all other Americans, are free to determine where and how they work, and to the significance of this freedom of choice for inducing changes in the ongoing system of medical care.

Part Three is concerned with the ever-larger role played by allied health manpower in meeting the rapidly increasing demands for more professionals and technicians. Particular note is taken of the potentialities and, even more, the limitations of the leadership of specific occupational groups in rationalizing their training systems and altering employment practices so that their members can work more effectively and receive higher compensation.

Part Four is concerned with illuminating the problems of persons suffering from chronic conditions and the extent to which their medical needs are intertwined with the socioeconomic structures in which they live and work. If the end of therapy is improved functioning, then indeed the physician's potential accomplishment is limited by the capacity of the society to provide a constructive place in which the chronically handicapped person can live and work.

In the concluding section an effort is made to point up the lessons that can be extracted from the last twenty-five years of the nation's efforts to improve its system of medical care and to relate these lessons to the challenges that lie ahead.

Money and trained manpower are scarce resources and additional inputs into the system of medical care must be thoughtfully planned and implemented; otherwise there will be little improvement in the health services provided, particularly for those sectors of the population who have the greatest need for more and better care. Although humanitarian sentiments and public funds exercise an influence on the distribution of medical services, their ability to modify the forces of the market place should not be exaggerated: regardless, the well-to-do will always be in a strong position to command most of the preferred services and most physicians will be more interested in serving them than in caring for the poor. Finally, physicians have strategic power to determine the speed and direction which the reform of the present system of medical care will take, and they will continue to have that power as long as the majority of Americans are reasonably satisfied with the medical care they receive.

It is one thing to design an improved system on paper; it is quite another to implement it. As we are learning in so many other sectors of American life—in racial matters, education, urban affairs, accident control—legislation is often able to bring about change but, alone it is seldom able to transform entrenched institutions that continue to command the tolerance, even the respect, of the majority of the population. The rate of change is usually determined by the order of dissatisfaction of the majority. That is the nature of a democracy.

PART ONE
Medicine and
the Economy

❧ 2 ❧

Facts and Fancies
About Medical Care

These have been brave new years. Our political leaders
have promised to eliminate poverty, abolish racial discrimination, provide educational opportunities for all, remove
substandard housing, vitalize our decaying cities, and enhance the national health by assuring access to quality
medical care for the groups who need it most—the poor and
the aged.

Only the innocent still believe that poverty, racial discrimination, inferior education, inadequate housing, and
urban blight will soon vanish from the face of the United
States. The gap between promise and accomplishment is
plainly visible to all. But with regard to medical care, the
situation is somewhat different. The radical new federal
health legislation is sufficiently recent that the intrinsic
shortcomings of the system have not yet become apparent.
In addition, the numerous and articulate proponents of
medical reform have been gratified with the interim success of three decades of persistent effort to reshape American medicine and they are optimistic about the future.
Medicare does provide protection against high hospital

and medical bills for most older persons who are caught
between increasing costs and fixed incomes. Medicaid has
made it much easier for welfare clients and some of the
medically indigent to avail themselves of a wider range of
health services. Act after act has been passed to expand the
supply of medical manpower, and initial steps have been
taken to improve health planning.

Medical planners will be the first to admit that many
more changes must be introduced before the system is fully
reconstructed. There is need to expand group-practice
units, to broaden comprehensive prepayment plans, to relate ambulatory to in-patient services, and to control quality.
The leaders are particularly concerned about the rapid increases in costs that show no signs of abating. But they are
confident that after years of frustration they have broken
the back of AMA reaction, and soon additional measures
will be enacted that will extend to every American the
benefits of quality medical care without financial strain.
Their optimism stems from convictions about our society,
our economy, and the health industry. Since only a mis-
anthrope would challenge the goals of reform, these convictions have seldom been subjected to critical analysis.
However, unless one adopts a critical stance toward goals,
resources, and mechanisms, sound progress will not be
made in the health field. Ten classic propositions that together comprise the decalogue of medical reform are here
subjected to critical review and evaluation.

1. *Medical care is unique in that it involves life-or-death.*
This is unquestionably true—but life-or-death is involved
in a minute fraction of all medical services rendered. For

the person who has been run down by a truck or has been shot, the speed with which he is transferred to a hospital and is operated upon may well determine whether he lives or dies. But it is a distortion of reality to see medical care primarily in this dramatic light.

An alternatve formulation would be that if the newborn is healthy, as is generally the case, and if he has healthy forebears, he is likely to grow up with little attention from physicians beyond routine pediatric services. In the absence of an inflamed appendix or some trauma, he (women of child-bearing age are excepted) may have only casual contact with the health services industry until he begins to decline, at which point medical specialists may have little objective help to offer him.

One of the socially useful functions of modern medicine is rehabilitation which enhances the adaptive level of an increasing number of the chronically ill and disabled. The individual who has a chronic impairment may live better, may remain useful and productive longer; however, his pathology can seldom be cured and his disabilities are seldom reversible.

Despite the substantial increases in expenditures for medical care, there has been no significant increase in male longevity during the past decade. Thus, unless man learns how to improve on the biblical standard of threescore-and-ten (with an additional decade for the righteous), medical care will remain what it has always been, largely supportive and ameliorative.

To put it differently, disease itself is largely self-limiting. People who are ill, even seriously ill, will generally get well without the active intervention of a physician. And more often than not, the conscientious physician will reassure the patient about his eventual recovery and do little or nothing but defer to nature. If the medical profession is ever moved to undertake a basic self-appraisal, it would be important to study the histories of patients with similar symptoms and conditions in terms of the interventions to which they were subjected. It is just possible that with regard to a wide range of conditions those who were treated least made the best progress.

2. *Improved medical care is the key to better health.* This is the assumption on which rests the long-time agitation for an improved system of medical care. But even the laity has recently indicated some skepticism about the limits of this assumption which underlay the huge congressional appropriations for medical research in the recent past. Recognizing that major progress was contingent upon new knowledge, the legislators have, since the early 1950s, favored expanded medical research over improved medical services in the competition for health funds. In the last years of the Johnson administration, executive policy shifted toward a correction of the balance in the direction of enhanced delivery of medical care, a reflection of mounting impatience with the limited applications of liberally financed research.

Additional parameters, however, must be introduced to set the true scope and limitations of the health services industry. We all know, though we tend to forget, that clean water and clean food and other environmental defenses have made the greatest contributions to raising the levels of health and decreasing the death rate. But we have been unable and unwilling to build on this history. Modern preventive medicine would force society to control automotive speeds since motor vehicle accidents are the single most important cause of death among the young and a major source of severe disability. Serious efforts to reduce the consumption of cigarettes would be undertaken. For the first time in our history more people die prematurely because they eat too much rather than too little.[1] Too much alcohol, too many drugs, and promiscuous sexual relations also take heavy tolls. On these fronts we are making little or no headway. In fact, we are probably retrogressing. Therapeutic medicine is not relevant, and effective preventive measures remain to be designed.

Too little income to buy adequate amounts and quality of food, to rent or own living quarters that are not decayed or decaying, to participate meaningfully in community activities, in work or learning programs, continues to be the most serious pathogen attacking the rural poor and the urban poor, the aged, and minority groups. Admittedly people with inadequate incomes also suffer from inadequate medical care, but improved nutrition and housing might contribute more to their health and longevity than easier access to physicians and hospitals. Many citizens would surely benefit from more and better medical care. But socioeconomic factors and the limitations of current scientific knowledge present real bounds to the promise of additional medical services leading to improved health.

3. *Improved medical care is a productive investment.* The last years have seen a reformulation of economics to

include investment in human beings within the main corpus. In an effort to explain the forces responsible for continuing and substantial increases in productivity, economists began to emphasize improvements in the quality of labor, particularly through education and health. Increased public and private expenditures for health were said to pay off in enhanced productivity.

Whatever the validity of this approach for developing countries with their high rates of mortality and morbidity —and even in these the result is uncertain because the survival of greater numbers may press against a limited food supply—its applicability to the United States is questionable. Unless it can be shown how more money for medical care will minimize respiratory diseases, the major cause of absenteeism; or alcoholism, a destroyer of talent; or heart disease and cancer, the principal causes of death in middle life; or accidents, which take a heavy toll among youth— unless larger expenditures for medical care can reduce these causes of morbidity and mortality, they cannot be justified as effective inputs for improved productivity, however desirable they may be for humanitarian and social reasons.

4. *Quality medical care is a right.* How can one question this proposition, especially if one recalls the AMA's long-term adherence to the contention that good medical care is a privilege? It is antediluvian to hold that economic resources should determine a man's eligibility for the benefits of modern medicine which, though infrequently, may mean the difference between life and death. But restiveness with a theory that emphasizes the consumer's dollars

as determinants of effective demand does not validate the other extreme, that quality medical care is a right inherent in citizenship.

Access to emergency care should be universally and unqualifiedly available, but this is not the issue here. Most medical care is not of this nature; it is more closely geared to alleviating pain and discomfort and providing reassurance and support. Yet lack of education, lack of income, lack of work, lack of suitable housing, lack of social acceptance because of the color of one's skin, and many other lacks also cause pain and discomfort—as much or more than does illness or disability. And we are still far from a national commitment that looks to the elimination of these sources of hurt and harm. Even as radical a social proposal as the negative income tax is considered in terms of an annual income of $3,200 per family of four, far short of $9,000, the U.S. Bureau of Labor Statistics figure (1967) for an adequate standard of living in a large city.

Generalizations about the right of every citizen to a high quality of medical care are easy to formulate, but they cannot be translated into policy until their proponents meet four preliminary tests: cost out the program; specify the sources of financing; present evidence that additional public efforts in this realm will yield benefits equal to or greater than if applied to other areas; and delineate how the services will in fact be provided.

5. *Other countries have a more efficient system of medical care.* Few nations have achieved more than half the per capita income of the United States. Yet it is contended that with limited resources many countries, notably Great

Britain, Soviet Russia, and the Scandinavian countries, have succeeded in developing systems of medical care which are superior to that of the United States. Special attention has been drawn to our rate of infant mortality and male longevity, which lag substantially behind those of many other Western countries.[2]

There is no possible justification for infant mortality rates to vary by some 400 percent within the borough of Brooklyn in New York City. Much of the difference must be ascribed to poor medical care. But we cannot ignore additional factors such as race, age, marital status, income, housing, and employment, which combine and interact to produce this shocking differential. Reworded, this means that the disturbingly high infant mortality rates found among Negroes and whites in low-income families reflect the wide economic and social gulfs that separate our urban and rural poor from the rest of the nation. None of the countries of Western Europe is confronted with such wide differences among classes and castes, and unless we succeed in eliminating the principal causes of these differences we probably will not be able to accomplish much by focusing solely on improving the structure of medical care.

The precise reasons for the shorter life expectancy of American middle-class white males remain obscure. Clearly there is more to the story than income. We suggested earlier that overeating tends to reduce longevity. And the same is probably true of excessive use of cigarettes and alcohol. But consumption patterns aside, there may be something else imbedded in the quality of contemporary life in the United States. The pace at which we work, travel, and play, and the frustrations that persist even in the face of a growing affluence, may hold the clue.

Key indices reveal not only that other countries lead the United States in national health standards, but they do so at a resource cost for medical care that is proportionately not higher than our own—and absolutely much less. In fact, it is so much less that we should be cautioned against assuming that much higher expenditures for medical care are likely to be reflected in lowered mortality. The simple fact is that the determinants of health are woven deep in the social fabric and that improvements in the system of medical care are likely to have only small impact.

6. *The competitive market is a poor instrument for allocating medical resources and distributing medical care.* We have already acknowledged that it would be irresponsible on both humanitarian and political grounds to deny emergency services to an individual simply because he cannot pay. The regrettable fact is that occasionally we do just that, although the instances are declining. Actually, we have never relied exclusively on the consumer to pay for health services. Philanthropy and government have long paid a part of the health bill, and in recent decades nonprofit insurance has played an increasingly important role in the financing of hospital care. Medicare and Medicaid are the most recent large-scale innovations aimed at increasing the purchasing power of the poor to obtain health services.

Assuming that improved medical care is desirable and that the provision of additional good medical services requires investment of additional scarce resources, it follows that society must rely on some rationing principle to allocate these services. Large-scale governmental financing can shift the relative position of various groups in their access to medical services, but there is little or no prospect—no matter how much money government invests—of equalizing the claims of all citizens so that need, rather than income, determines the services rendered to each individual.

Rationing according to need would require that government control all of the strategic resources, particularly manpower. Only if the individual physician, nurse, and technician were subject to direct control could such a system be structured. After many years of effort, even the USSR is still far from this ideal. The discrepancy between the quantity and quality of medical services available in the city and in rural areas remains substantial. The same obtains in Great Britain and in every other country that has sought to establish a comprehensive system of medical care based on need.

The United States is a country of continental proportions historically committed to the doctrine of freedom of choice in work. Moreover, there are major differences in the distribution of income among regions and within regions, among families and individuals. And our heterogeneous population encompasses racial and ethnic groups that have been only partially incorporated into the dominant society. Given these overriding geographic, economic, and demographic variables, any serious proposal to establish a more equitable system of medical care within our present society has no prospect of success unless profound structural alterations occur in our free-market economy.

First, government's financial inputs on behalf of the poor

would have to be extremely large. Simultaneously, competitive bidding for medical services by the upper- and middle-income classes would have to cease or at least abate substantially. And finally, decision-making by critical producers of services, particularly physicians, with regard to locus, field, and mode of practice would have to be governed exclusively by prospective dollar income. With none of these changes even remotely possible, augmented purchasing power in the hands of the poor cannot effect any significant redistribution of medical services.

To continue the argument a step further. If supply creates its own demand—and there is strong evidence that this is true at least for certain types of medical services—then no amount of money that government would appropriate for this purpose would eliminate the necessity of rationing services. This being the case, the most reasonable system would involve rigorous adherence to priorities based on objectively determined need. But when have human systems been known to obey the laws of logic? As the English experience has shown, once old people with chronic illness have been admitted to the hospital, it is not easy to transfer them to another facility when it has been determined that they can no longer profit from general hospital care. Consequently there is a long waiting list for elective surgery. A leading teaching hospital in a major American city finds that it can admit patients who require surgery for carcinoma only after some three weeks, so tight are its facilities. A high proportion of its beds are occupied by patients who can probably profit from further care but whose need is considerably less than those who wait. Still, allocation by medical priority does not occur. One way of interpreting the evidence is to infer that the community has too few general hospital beds or perhaps too few beds in nursing homes. But this particular city has the highest concentration of medical resources per capita of any community in the United States!

Dissatisfaction with the competitive market is justified. Its worst effects can surely be mitigated by judicious interferences. But to contend that it is only a question of more federal money or the introduction of a comprehensive system of medical insurance that stands in the way of providing adequate medical care to all citizens is social fantasy.

7. *Consumer satisfaction with medical care.* Economists have long recognized that the nub of a competitive system is one in which the consumer decides how to spend his money. He determines whether one good or service is better than another at or near the same price, and he backs his judgment with his money. To behave rationally the consumer must be competent, he must have access to market information, and he must be able to choose among competing products and producers.

However this model, as many economists recognize, is not adequate to the market for medical care. Even the intelligent and the educated are unable to make discriminatory judgments about a professional service except indirectly—that, is in terms of the producer's reputation, field of specialization, even age and fee; or retrospectively—in terms of outcome: did the patient recover? Without relevant information and criteria for evaluation, the layman is in a poor position to judge the quality of medical care.

What then determines consumer behavior and satisfaction? The patient at least knows whether he likes a physician. Since often the care he seeks and receives is essentially reassurance and support, he can obtain these best from a physician with whom he establishes rapport. Frequently he relies on the recommendation of relatives or friends, whose assessment is based on prior experience. The more sophisticated purchaser may apply certain objective criteria: whether the physician is board-certified, his hospital affiliations, and similar insignia.

Physicians, as any group of professionals, differ. Some are concerned with optimizing their income. Others are determined to practice medicine according to the standards which they have been taught and to which they adhere. Most effect a compromise: they want a good income and they want to practice good medicine. But they know that the consumer (with money to spend) chooses among physicians.

While good hospitals can effectively govern the quality of medicine and surgery practiced within their halls, there is little peer control on the outside where traditional ethics constrain physicians to maintain silence about another's work. As a consequence, many consumers spend a great amount of money in the search for cures that cannot be found; others have unnecessary operations; and more than a few lose their lives as a result of faulty diagnosis and inept intervention. Every major hospital counts among its patients a minority who are there because they have previously been poorly treated, often very poorly. Some patients never have the opportunity for a second time.

Since this is the manner in which the system of medical care operates, one might assess again the gains that would accrue from facilitating consumer-choice of physician. Those who consider Medicaid as an unalloyed boon might consider all the implications of transferring medical care of the poor out of its traditional site, the clinics of teaching hospitals, at least in large eastern cities, into the open market of private practice. It is not at all certain that the gain in dignity and self-esteem to the welfare patient who is now capable of paying a private physician would outweigh the loss in quality of care that might ensue by his transferring from the hospital clinic to the physician's office.

Without contending that physicians are greedy or that most patients are hypochondriacal, we should admit that the chief deterrents to overtreatment are the current tautness in physician supply (which enables the practitioner to reduce the number of visits per patient to a minimum at no loss of income to himself) and the fee-for-service payment system (a major consumer constraint). In any attempt at restructuring the medical care system, it is important to remember that it is the physician who determines whether the patient is to be seen again and that there is a significant minority of patients who, given the opportunity, would tend to preempt a considerable portion of the physician's time. This suggests that when the government pays the bill, physicians have great latitude in determining the level of their income and that no expansion of the supply of physicians is likely to enable them to meet the emotional needs of that segment of the population who are anxious about their health.

A critical limitation of the consumer's ability to assess objectively the quality of the care which he receives is a function of the fact that much of the physician's efficacy rests upon his ability to develop a rapport with his patient. While psyche and soma can interact to produce subjective improvement, this is not necessarily the same as relieving the patient of the pathological causes of his symptomatology. A modern system of medical care cannot rest on consumer satisfaction any more than it can rely on the discipline of the medical profession. Here, as elsewhere, reasonable rather than optimum solutions will have to suffice.

8. *Medical manpower is in short supply.* No single position is so widely or firmly held at present than the assumption that the principal difficulties on the American medical scene reflect a shortage of critical types of specialized manpower, particularly physicians, nurses, and technicians. Even the AMA, after years of voicing vehement opposition followed by years of neutrality, has now joined the choir of voices advocating a rapid and sustained increase in the number of physicians. And almost everyone concerned, from patient to physician, has long bemoaned the shortage of registered nurses.

What are the facts and how can we interpret them? Those who contend that there is a physician shortage resort to various ratios between the number of active practitioners and the total population. When these data revealed that there had been no slippage over the last quarter century but even a slight improvement (depending on the base year selected), attention shifted to the census of physicians in private practice or of those who are in general family practice, as distinct from specialists. This usually produced the looked-for statistical result.

None of the analysts has taken into account that the radical shift toward specialization must be associated with substantive improvements in the structure of medical care, and that it is a travesty to use manpower criteria based on utilization patterns of the 1930s to judge adequacy in the late 1960s. Moreover, factors contributing to enhanced utilization of physicians' time, such as the decline of home visits in favor of office and hospital services, have usually been omitted from these calculations. In addition, the statisticians paid little attention to the spectacular development of paramedical manpower, which has grown much more rapidly than almost any other group in the entire economy. As a final resort, the advocates of the shortage argument have insisted that the radical expansion in per capita demand for physician services must be taken into account. A public that wants to spend more money for physicians' services either directly or through taxes is surely entitled to do so, they say, and it is the responsibility of the public and professional leadership to assure that the required personnel is educated and available. The last point has particular relevance with regard to the nursing profession, where all the ratios between registered and practical nurses and nurse's aides and the population show large increases.

Beginning with the Magnuson Report in the early 1950s, one impressive commission after another has added its voice to urgent requests for more medical manpower. However, the most recent to report—the National Advisory Commission on Health Manpower (1967)—has finally taken a more searching view. After giving recognition to the many recent voluntary efforts toward the further expansion of medical education, the report questions whether additional large-scale federal action to speed the process would necessarily be in the public interest unless other changes were introduced antecedently or concomitantly to improve significantly the utilization of the existing medical manpower which now numbers between 3 and 4 million persons.

It would not be fair to suggest that the Commission opposes measures aimed at increasing the supply. But it is the first public body to recognize that even rapid increases in the supply might have only a minimal effect upon the total system without radical and fundamental changes in the organization and delivery of medical services.

To put it simply: To increase the output of medical schools in New York State, or even in New York City, by 10 percent in the next four years would not guarantee that more physicians would be available to treat the ghetto poor. And it would be even more naive to assume that an increased output of the medical schools in New Orleans or Birmingham would result in more physicians practicing in the Delta.

It has been suggested that medical care may represent an unusual situation in which the supply creates the demand. It follows that accelerating further the supply of medical manpower (in which the rate of employment from 1950-65 has grown at about five times the rate for the nation at

large) holds little promise of eliminating shortages. New
criteria must be introduced to assess the number and quality of medical personnel in whose preparation and employment society should invest.

9. *The AMA is responsible for most of the shortcomings
in the prevailing system of medical care.* It would be difficult to find a professional or trade association that has more
consistently or more vigorously supported the wrong side
of every public issue in which it had a major stake than the
AMA. For a long time the leaders of organized medicine
obstructed the establishment of prepaid group practice
units; until recently they were opposed to the expansion of
medical education; to this day they have successfully re-
sisted federal subsidization of medical education with the
result that entrance into the profession is blocked for most
young Americans whose parents do not have ample income.
The AMA fought the passage of Medicare every step of the
way, and when it capitulated it insisted that the law provide reimbursement to physicians on a fee-for-service basis,
which may or may not prove to be tenable—and the latter
is more likely. Recently it passed resolutions opposing the
innovative techniques undertaken by the Office of Economic Opportunity to bring health services to the poor. In
addition to blocking practically every effort to modify the
existing market structure for medical care, it has moved
slowly to provide leadership in such vital areas as improving controls over the quality of medical care that the
American people are receiving.

Despite these indictments—and the list of commissions
and omissions could be extended—it is an error to contend

that the present structure of American medicine would be vastly different were it not for the conservative stance of the AMA.

Every group in the United States is dedicated to advancing its own special interests; usually their goals are held to be consonant with the national interest. This holds for the military, business, university professors, lawyers—every organized group. There is no reason to expect physicians to act otherwise.

The AMA has adopted and supported policies which the majority of its membership expects will provide physicians with the optimal conditions for practice, which are defined in terms of self-determination and self-regulation. No profession willingly cedes part of its independence; by definition, a professional man is able to determine how best to employ his talents and skill.

The physicians, who number only about 300,000 out of a total health work force of some 4 million, play and will continue to play a pivotal role in the organization and functioning of the entire system of medical care. But a similar pattern obtains in other professional fields. Professors determine the functioning of the university; the senior military usually have the deciding voice in defense policy; public school teachers and administrators determine the style and content of public education; the behavior of members of the bar determines the quality of legal services. And each group insists that it operates in the public interest.

Before we can conclude that the AMA alone is responsible for most of the shortcomings of the prevailing structure of medical care, let us consider some other facts. Hospitals have come to occupy an ever more important role in the provision of critical medical services, and most hospitals are under the control of voluntary organizations whose lay leaders are formally and legally invested with policy-making powers. If hospitals do not operate effectively, the trustees bear the ultimate responsibility. No one familiar with the hospital scene will deny that most trustees are poorly qualified to exercise their responsibilities and, in fact, most do not.

To sharpen the issue: One criticism of our present system of hospital care relates to the large numbers of foreign-trained (i.e., inadequate) physicians on house staffs. However, without them, many hospitals would have no physician on duty from 6 P.M. until 8 A.M. It would require only a modest amount of acumen and firmness for a hospital board to institute mandatory night duty for the visiting staff in return for the privilege of using the hospital's facilities for their private patients. Such a system operates in certain small communities, but it is not the general pattern.

Nor can we ignore established consumer behavior. Many persons would be willing to forego the privilege of choosing their own physician if they had assurance that an alternative system of medical care would provide optimal service. But there are many others to whom the free choice of physician is not a whim but a basic right for which they are willing to pay, even dearly. This is easily proved by the number of middle-income members of various prepayment plans who choose to go outside the plan when they must undergo surgery and pay the fees of a nonaffiliated surgeon.

Further, third parties, such as government, Blue Cross, commercial insurance, and labor–management groups, are heavily involved in the purchase of medical care. Not every third party acts with fiduciary and social responsibility to see that the dollars it spends for health are used effectively.

In our social and economic system, in which each organized group operates in the interest of its members, we cannot single out the AMA as the major villain. Although the leaders of organized medicine have failed to lead, so have the leaders of hospitals (governmental and nonprofit), of health agencies, of business and trade unions that are major purchasers, and of other strategic groups, including the progressive leaders of medical education who have recently been singled out as the executors of all the unfinished business of medical reform.

10. *Better planning is the answer.* The growing concern with the large-scale and sustained rise in medical costs has led more and more persons, in and out of government, to look at the present system of medical care in the hope of identifying how present and prospective resources could be better deployed and more effectively utilized. As early as the 1930s experiments in regionalization were initiated. It was assumed that if the local physician could be tied into the local general hospital, and if the local general hospital could be effectively related to a large specialized center, costs could be controlled and the quality of services improved. Military medicine operates on this principle and with considerable success. But the military controls both the patient and the physician. Since no organization in

civilian life exercises comparable control, the reformers have been pressing for an improved system of planning based on incentives and sanctions.

Within narrow limits we can point to some modest successes of regional planning and integration of historically autonomous services. We might even anticipate further successes in the years ahead as a result of the deeper financial involvement of government and pressure from various groups in the population who are deprived of access to quality care or who find it difficult to meet the steeply mounting costs.

But some questions arise. Agreement among voluntary and governmental agencies working in the same arena is difficult to achieve. The concern of medical schools with teaching and research are not readily reconcilable with the desire of the urban and rural poor for greater access to routine medical services. There is a chasm between public health agencies and hospitals that has seldom been bridged.

But the nub of the difficulty lies deeper than the institutional level. In small- and medium-sized communities, most physicians in active practice have a hospital affiliation, and there is no split between insiders and outsiders. But this is not true of many large hospital centers with closed staffs, which frequently employ physicians on salary. Effective planning in large communities comes face to face with basic economics. Why should a physician on the outside turn over "his" patient to an insider? And how can the hospital be restructured to serve as the fulcrum for an improved system of medical care unless there is a place on the hospital's staff for every physician in the community to share in its work and its income?

There are a limited number of communities in this large country where a new and improved system of relating patients to physicians and physicians to hospitals has been instituted. But the successful experiments are still few, and almost every one reflects the presence of a special factor—outstanding professional leadership or financial subsidy by business or government.

The presumption is that planning will continue and that it will chalk up modest victories, but there is little prospect under the present realities of a free society and a free economy that the major participants from physicians to patients will be able to move far or fast to reshape the existing system significantly through planning. And relying on medical schools to assume effective leadership, as the reformers do, is an act of faith, not reason. Historically, no major institution has been more estranged from the community and its concerns than the university, and new constructive relationships will at best come slowly.

It has not been difficult to raise objections to the conventional wisdom about medical care and its overdue reformation. But it would be unsporting not to propose a modest alternative approach to the desideratum of improved health care. In place of an unrealistic brave new world in which all the shortcomings of the present system are to disappear in short order by new methods of planning, organization, financing, and control, a limited number of modest priority objectives have been singled out together with summary suggestions as to how they might conceivably be implemented.

The scarcity of medical services for the rural population cannot be eliminated, but it can be alleviated through the development of state and federal scholarships for medical students given with the proviso that upon graduation the young doctors will accept appointment for a limited period, say three years or so, in a rural area, preferably near an area hospital. Since experience with this approach has had a mixed record, we should also place reliance on a program of upgrading public health nurses to serve as primary medical screener-therapists in isolated areas. Patients with complications would be referred by these nurses to the nearest hospital with ambulatory as well as inpatient services. The charge that this would leave rural America underdoctored is admitted. The important question here is whether this approach of relying on a nurse-screener-therapist-educator offers a prospect of modest progress.

The urban poor have also encountered difficulties in obtaining proper medical attention, but their presence and pressure have stimulated the development within teaching hospitals of comprehensive outpatient departments and the expansion of emergency-room services. The present tendency to deprecate these facilities is wrong. Instead, emphasis should be placed on strengthening them and making them more efficient and effective. They hold the best promise of providing care for the urban poor.

Second, rather than seeking to attract private physicians into the ghetto or devising ways of enabling the poor to buy services outside of their area, it might prove more sensible to attach to each urban hospital a corps of nurses specially trained to visit families at home for the purpose of screening and referral and once again to serve as health educators.

The third approach would be to improve the diagnostic, referral, and follow-up mechanisms of school health programs in poor neighborhoods so that children with medical problems, which might otherwise remain neglected, can be identified and appropriate therapeutic and rehabilitative procedures initiated.

Such an approach offers the urban poor, like the rural poor, much less than has been ideally proposed, but more than they now have and even more than they are likely to have under ambitious programs such as Medicaid, or with elaborate community health centers which may never be able to mobilize the monetary and manpower resources they require.

Next to improving medical care for the rural and urban poor, the major challenge is to prevent middle-income groups from suffering severe financial hardships as a result of illness or disability. The best prospect of making significant progress toward this objective would be new and improved programs of major medical insurance with reasonable deductibles and co-insurance. Let us be clear. Short of a compulsory system of national health insurance, and probably not even then, there is no way to provide all citizens with complete prepaid coverage for all their medical needs. Nor is there any need, unless one takes seriously the claims —and these have never been adequately documented—that much ill health among lower-income groups is attributable to a lack of preventive services together with the failure of these groups to seek therapeutic services because of the cost. There is merit to these claims, but we do not know how much.

The quality of medical care for rich and poor alike is far below what it could be if the profession and government introduced more systematic efforts to monitor the services that are provided in hospitals and in the community. The challenge, however, is to achieve greater comprehension by all parties—the public, the politicians, and the physicians— of the right of laymen to such protection and the social gains that would accrue. Here is one major line of reform where the prospective costs are small, the prospective gains large. The range of instruments is wide, from statistical reporting and evaluation through continuing education for doctors and greater efforts to associate every practicing physician with a general hospital. More contentious devices, such as periodic re-examination for licensure, can be held in abeyance until more acceptable reforms have been instituted and evaluated.

It is generally agreed that the present utilization of medical resources is poor because of the perverse ways in which medical services are produced and distributed. To mention three outstanding shortcomings: community planning and individual hospital management are weak; hospital insurance that is limited to inpatient services tends to inflate costs; and fee-for-service is the most costly method of physician reimbursement. Unless key groups, such as third parties who purchase care and hospital trustees, exercise leadership to improve planning and management, there is little prospect that total medical expenditures can be brought under control. We may be on the way to raising our total annual outlays from $50 billion to $100 billion within less than one decade, with little likelihood of getting much more or much better care than we do now.

Clearly we need innovation in insurance so that coverage can be extended to include diagnostic work performed on ambulatory patients. The experiments now under way need to be increased and evaluated, and if the results are favorable new policies should be forthcoming.

Finally, we have had sufficient experience in the last few years to be on guard against infusing new money into the system without exacting a return. Money is leverage and it should be used to extract concessions from the major interest groups so that the prevailing system can slowly be rationalized. Otherwise we will pour more and more money into a system that is characterized by consumer ignorance, a seller's monopoly, inefficiency, lack of accountability—all of which can lead only to further dissipation of resources.

The medical reformer will have disdain for the modest proposals set out above. He will emphasize that the major shortcomings that now characterize the medical care of American citizens will not be eliminated, not even substantially reduced, even if all of the proposals were put into effect. This is granted. But they have been put forward on the following premise: There is no way of equalizing the share of the poor in high quality, privately produced American medicine (the so-called "mainstream"), and we should therefore attempt to improve the services to which they have access. There is no way of removing the financial hurdles to quality medical care for families with modest incomes, but the expansion of major medical insurance could help. There is no way of using additional public and private resources intelligently unless the planning, organization, and management of the system is improved, and this can come about only as the public, the politicians, and the physicians understand the issues and are willing to act. We cannot speedily devise a good system of medical care for all even if we were willing to pay the price.

There is a great deal that is wrong with the prevailing system of medical care in the United States. But this is true of every other major aspect of our national life—education, housing, employment, urban communities, race relations. Democracy means that the rate of reform is determined by the level of discontent of the majority. It does not appear that the American public is ready or nearly ready to abolish the existing system of medical care. Surely the physicians are not. And no politician is offering a radically new program. It looks as if we will be forced to muddle ahead. Even to muddle, we need to be responsive to facts, not fancies.

~ 3 ~

The Health Services Industry

In recent years, much has been made of the "shortage" of medical manpower, of a "crisis" in the medical field. In this country the word "crisis" is used too freely. The United States is rich; we are rich in people, skills, refrigerators, automobiles. But those who have a little want more, and those who have a great deal also want more. In such a situation it matters little that we are rich, or even very rich, in comparison with other people and other lands. The point is that here *at home* there is a gap between what we have and what we want. We are chronically short of all the good things of which we want more.

The dynamic nature of our economy and society helps to create the very shortages about which we complain, some of which we have not been able to overcome despite long and continuing efforts. For example, the federal government and other agencies together with the American consumer are now spending much more money in the health field than they used to spend. Presumptively this means that they are now obtaining more and better health services than a few years ago. We must emphasize the term "presumptively," however, for with the rapid rise in prices the additional dollars may reflect primarily a more liberal reward to the participating factors of production. But if the perspective is broadened to include a longer sweep of time, we know this is not the whole, or even the largest, part of the story because there has been a marked per capita increase in manpower and other resources devoted to health and medical services.

The health services industry has in fact been remarkably responsive to the demand for expansion. In manpower terms the industry increased by over 50 percent in the decade of the 1950s; add the years 1960-1966, and the total gain exceeds 90 percent. It has been one of our fastest growing industries. There is certainly some basis for concern with the current and long-run imbalances between the demand and supply in certain categories of scarce medical manpower, but the field as a whole has demonstrated substantial flexibility.

In 1940, the health sector preempted 3 percent of all nonagricultural employment; in 1960, the proportion was 5 percent. The absolute figures, 1 million in 1940, 2.6 million in 1960, and an estimated 3 million in 1966, indicate even more dramatically the response of the health services field to the rapidly increasing demand.

Before considering the specific characteristics of the health services field, let us review the broad dimensions of the service sector of the economy, of which health services are one important part. It is important to note that 2 out of every 3 workers in the United States are employed in the service sector rather than in the goods-producing sector. Further, the services tend to use a greater proportion of highly trained persons than does the goods-producing sector.

Since more and more scientific and technical manpower is centered in the services, the future progress of the economy is increasingly dependent upon the education and training of the prospective members of the labor force. A man without a solid educational foundation will find it increasingly difficult to acquire a high order of skill. Moreover, unless a man has access to continuing education and training, the skills which he has acquired are likely to obsolesce. Critical linkages have come to exist among the growth of the services, broadened access to educational and training opportunities, and a trained manpower supply.

The health services industry should be particularly sensitive and responsive to matters of education and training, since it must recruit large numbers of people to cover both its present and prospective requirements. In addition, the more specialized the education a person acquires, the more likely he is to remain attached to the field that he enters. Of course, this proposition must be handled with caution when it is applied to certain types of professionals, such as engineers and lawyers, since many of them, despite their professional education, do not remain in their profession but move into business, politics, or administration. But the proposition has general validity.

The service field is characterized by a high proportion of women workers. Women workers have certain characteristics: on the average they tend to acquire somewhat less education and training than do men; many who work prefer to work part time or part year; and they have distinctive patterns of entering, leaving, and returning to the labor force. There are other ways in which women differ from men with respect to their preparation for and participation in the labor force, including the age when they study, the fields they enter, and their attachment to their occupation. An employer cannot afford to ignore these important differences, especially if women comprise a large part of his labor force.

Until recently trade unions have been underrepresented in the service sector of the economy. We are now beginning to see a shift. They still tend to be underrepresented in the nonprofit or governmental sector. However, changes loom ahead. One can speculate that the trade-union strength in the future may be centered in the not-for-profit sector. Today, more and more governmental agencies have agreed that their employees can join unions, even if most of these agreements carry a no-strike clause. However, when bargaining breaks down between the parties, when serious disagreements cannot be resolved, these no-strike clauses tend to be ignored. New York State has long had a law on its books preventing public employees from striking, and violation of this law carries severe penalties. But we have had a series of strikes in New York by public employees in which, after settlement was reached, the penalties have usually been waived. The simple fact is that in most instances the penalty of dismissal would not provide the relief that the governmental employer needs or desires.

In many service fields, nonprofessional workers tend to have low wages, poor working conditions, and a limited range of fringe benefits. This reflects many different forces, including the lack of union strength in the nonprofit sector in which many service workers are employed. An additional reason for the lower wages and the less attractive working conditions in many parts of the service sector is the difficulty of increasing productivity which usually makes it possible to pay workers more.

As noted earlier, the services tend to make use of a relatively high proportion of professional workers. Now the nature of professional work makes it difficult to set output norms and even more difficult to establish and control the work flow. Moreover, professionals balk at close supervision. The scope for managerial initiative is constricted. It is next to impossible, for instance, for a university president or a dean to introduce a series of organizational changes that will lead to a greater utilization of academic resources, particularly faculty time and effort. This would require years of subtle negotiation since a faculty believes that it should control its own work.

Against the background of these general characteristics of the service sector, let us look more closely at the health services industry from the viewpoint of its manpower requirements and the problems that it faces in seeking to meet them.

The first point is that the manpower required to provide services usually must be located close to or in the immediate proximity of the place where the services are to be consumed. This means that while certain members of the health services industry may be more or less mobile, most of the workers must be recruited from the locale where the physician's office, the public health clinic, or the hospital is located. Since a high proportion of all health workers cannot be effectively employed until they have had some specialized education and training, the training structures must be distributed throughout the country so that potential workers have access to them. Otherwise, those who are able and willing to enter the health field will not be able to, and those who seek trained and competent workers will be unable to find them.

Whether the health services industry is able to fill its jobs depends, of course, on more than the availability of local training facilities, crucial as these are. At the same time that clinics and hospitals are looking for workers to train and hire or hire and train, so are many competing employers. The prospective employee, in deciding upon a field, considers not only the time and other costs of pursuing training, but also the wages and working conditions that he can look forward to once he has been trained. For many different reasons, imbedded in the history of the industry, its methods of financing and the nature of its management, the wage structure in health services, at least at the subprofessional level, continues to lag behind other fields. This fact complicates its recruiting problem.

Another reason that the industry faces difficulties in maintaining an adequate supply of trained manpower is its heavy dependence on female labor, particularly young women, who characteristically have a high rate of withdrawal from the labor force. In addition, many workers leave for other types of employment where the wages and working conditions are better. Consequently the health services industry has long had a high replacement demand at the same time that it has sought additional staff to cover its expansion needs.

The industry's difficulties, with respect to both attraction and retention, have been further complicated by the fact that so many workers sooner or later discover that they have little opportunity to advance. Many workers would be willing to accept initially low wages or adverse working conditions if they could look to a brighter future. This is in fact the situation of the young physician during his years of internship and residency. He is willing to accept the modest stipend and adjust to an arduous working schedule because he knows that he can look forward to much higher earnings and improved conditions. But such favorable prospects are not part of the career expectations of the nurse, the dietitian, or the medical technician. In few fields are the ceilings so low. There is little opportunity for the ambitious and capable person to advance through performance on the job. If he wants to better himself he must return to school and start off on a new track which will land him at a higher point in the hierarchy. But this is too costly in terms of time and money for most to contemplate.

A structured training system, however, can be a major attraction in personnel procurement and retention if it is closely aligned to both the wage structure and to the promotion ladder. The Armed Services discovered that they could help alleviate the shortages of skilled manpower which they confronted by establishing more attractive career opportunities to encourage men to reenlist: they offered training programs which would qualify the men for the higher paying and more prestigious positions. But the health services industry has not yet succeeded in doing this. Even within the hospital it is difficult to get the several independent professional and technical groups to take steps which would make it easier for persons lower on the ladder to qualify for better positions and be promoted into them.

The federal government is now committed to alleviating health manpower shortages. However, its ability to do so should not be overestimated. For example, the Nurse Training Act of 1964 committed the federal government to spend large sums for the training of nurses. One careful student of the subject, after reviewing the initial experience under the Act, ventured the judgment that the result of the federal effort might have been a net reduction in the supply.[1]

The hospital has long played a crucial role in the training of health personnel, because among other reasons it needs to hire large numbers of unskilled workers from the local community who want to continue to work in the community. Despite this history, hospitals have never been able to perform an effective educational and training mission. They have been neither properly financed nor staffed. In fact, for a long time they were able to cover their training costs by extracting a large amount of unremunerated labor from physicians, nurses, technicians, and others. Recently, they have sought to recapture some of their training costs from Blue Cross and other third parties, but they have met substantial and growing resistance. The patient and the insurance carrier see little logic in assessing the sick and injured to pay the costs involved in training medical manpower. Clearly these training costs should be assessed against the community at large.

The fact that most types of specialized education and

training have been brought under the rubric of the formal educational system adds to the incongruity of continuing medical education and training by the hospital. While there has been some shift in the last years to include more health and medical training within the formal educational structure, the hospital continues to serve as a major center even though it is frequently ill equipped because of insufficient finances and staff to carry out these responsibilities efficiently and effectively.

The hospital, both as a training and as an employing institution, has made an imperfect adjustment to the revolution in manpower that has been under way in this country since World War II. During the last quarter-century, more and more married women have become interested in working out of the home. But for women to take hospital jobs, especially at higher levels of competence, often requires adjustments in the conditions and particularly the scheduling of the work. In this country, employment is structured to meet the needs of a characteristically male, youthful, unencumbered labor force, and has been slow in accommodating to the female, married, somewhat older worker. A clear case in point is seen in so traditionally female a field as nursing, where control of the profession had long been in the hands of single women careerists who looked askance at others less willing or able to become so deeply involved.

Another factor that has added to the manpower difficulties in the health field grows out of a chronic under-investment of capital. Manpower utilization is a function of the demands of the job in relation to the skills of the worker, the capital at his disposal, and the quality of the supervision which he receives. Many have questioned whether hospitals and other health agencies make efficient use of the people on their payroll. There is considerable evidence to suggest that they do not, because of both inadequate capital investment and poor supervision. Health agencies thus tend to use more people than they would otherwise require, and the dollars at their disposal must be spread thinner and each worker paid less. If the hospital operates with antiquated plant and equipment because the public is underinvesting, it is difficult to improve its manpower utilization.

A central challenge to every service field is to provide not only an adequate quantity of services but also services of quality. It is clear that we want teachers, ministers, physicians, and nurses who are competent. But every field must take care not to establish standards for their own sake. For example, nursing leaders have been seeking to attract more nurses with baccalaureate and master's and even doctor's degrees.

An influential segment has striven to establish the four-year college course as required training for staff nursing in place of the standard three-year in-hospital course. But hospital administrators have been buying a different type of bedside nursing personnel in the market. While there is no evident unemployment of nurses with high orders of formal education, hospital directors have been satisfied to provide the bulk of nursing services through modestly trained practical nurses and aides. There is no justification for elongating training requirements under the undefined rubric of quality with no corresponding differentiation of professional duties and functions.

While quality is of crucial importance in the provision of services, it often provides an umbrella for all sorts of machinations. Some years ago psychiatrists at the Menninger Foundation outlined the qualifications of a good ward attendant. They said that a man with an eighth-grade education, with a friendly personality, with a willingness to work with sick people, would make a better attendant than a college graduate who had majored in biology. Emotional characteristics often are more important than intellectual characteristics. A man with minimum education who can live in an environment made up of people who are mentally ill and can establish satisfying relations with the patients may be better qualified to work in a mental hospital than a highly educated person.

Another barrier to effective manpower utilization in the health field is the continuing struggle among the many professional and semiprofessional groups. All have a role to play in the provision of health and medical services, yet each devotes an inordinate amount of time and energy to improving its position on the ladder by seeking to move itself up a rung or two and in turn seeking to prevent those below from impinging on its rights and prerogatives. The struggle for market power and social prestige between physicians and nurses, between nurses and technicians, between technicians and aides, makes the design of a rational, long-term policy for manpower utilization next to impossible. People are motivated to work more and better by the prospects of improving themselves. Nevertheless, a newly graduated staff nurse receives substantially the same pay as a staff nurse with forty years of experience!

Now, the health services field alone does not have sufficient leverage to remedy chronic in-fighting. The people at the top do not want to change anything; the people at the bottom are too weak to change anything; those in between cannot agree on what should be changed and, if they did agree, they still would not have the power to bring about the desired changes.

But our society does have a way of accomplishing change in the face of recalcitrance and impotence of various groups. The market is a potent mechanism. When the supply of registered nurses proved inadequate, a new source of supply was opened up. Training programs for practical nurses were established and, over the opposition of the leaders of the nursing profession, many middle-aged women with limited education were attracted into the field Since today they are able to earn about 80 percent of what a general duty registered nurse can earn, at the end of one instead of three years of training, the likelihood is that the shift in the direction of a higher proportion of practical nurses will continue.

Similarly, although the leaders of psychiatry continue to insist that only qualified psychiatrists who have obtained their MD degrees can practice psychotherapy, many other disciplines provide training that appears to be adequate and is much shorter. Today many psychologists, social workers, ministers, and counselors are working successfully in the field of psychotherapy.

The problem of an adequate number of properly qualified medical manpower will probably never be solved, because the level of demand for medical services is in considerable measure determined by the supply. Whatever the level of supply, the demand will rise beyond it. We have lived, and we must continue to live, with manpower shortages. We must reconcile ourselves to this fact of life and recognize that there are better and worse ways to cope with shortages.

It does not follow, of course, that the shorter the period of training, the more effective the level of manpower utilization. But the foregoing does imply the danger of various professional groups seeking to establish requirements for training that are unrealistic since employers cannot attract the numbers required to provide the quantity of services that the public demands. It remains the responsibility of the leadership of the several professional organizations to strive to establish standards that will assure services of acceptable quality. But quality alone cannot become their sole preoccupation. Quantity is likewise a legitimate requirement in providing services for the mass of the population, one that must be met. The balancing of the two is the challenge to professional leadership.

We must use what some have called the "crisis" in medical manpower and what could perhaps better be designated as a "chronic situation" to learn more about the people who can be recruited and trained; preferred methods of training; the relationships of training to wage and career structures; the balancing of professional and group conflicts; and effective management and supervision.

❧ 4 ❧
Hospitals and Collective Bargaining

Something new is happening in the hospital field. Unions have begun to organize various groups of professional and nonprofessional hospital workers. To understand what is under way, to appreciate why unions are only now getting started, and to estimate what the future has in store, it would be helpful to take an analytical glance at the hospital as an economic institution.

Some Salient Facts About Hospitals

A few facts about the health services industry. The first is that the health services industry today is big industry, big money, big manpower. It accounts for expenditures of over $50 billion annually; it employs between 3 and 4 million people.[1]

The hospital is increasingly the key institution in the industry; construction costs included, it absorbs about 40 percent of the money. Within the hospital structure, 60 percent of all expenditures go for personnel.

Physicians play a key role in medical care. However, the manpower statistics by themselves do not make this clear. In an industry with a total labor force of between 3 and 4 million, there are only about 300,000 physicians. Quantitatively, physicians represent 10 percent or less of all medical workers.

Another striking aspect of the industry is that despite large incremental inputs of money, manpower, and other resources over the past two decades, the gap between what the public desires and what is available may be as wide as ever—if not wider. The American people appear to have a voracious appetite when it comes to consuming medical resources.

Still another facet of the industry is the high degree of professionalization and specialization of its manpower. Yet, once again, the statistics do not make this clear. A large proportion of all employees have less than a high-school education. The industry utilizes highly trained persons such as neurosurgeons, who require a decade or more to complete their medical training, but at the same time it utilizes many unskilled persons. While professionals play a key role in the provision of health services, they are in the minority; workers with less than a college education are in the majority.

When unskilled workers are hired by the hospital, they receive a little on-the-job training. Many of these workers are women, and women have a less close attachment to the labor market than do men. As a consequence, most hospitals have high turnover rates. Here is a major industry in which one model is a Nobel prize winner, but an equally apposite model is a young woman, a "high-school dropout," who is willing to work in a hospital until she can find a better job or a husband. In evaluating the health services industry we must balance between these two models.

Let us now look at the hospital structure more closely. There are over 7,000 hospitals of all types in the nation. In addition, there are about 12,000 nursing homes, and this number is likely to increase substantially in the near future.[1] Then there are a considerable number of free-standing health stations, clinics, and community health centers. Until recently the Office of Economic Opportunity looked forward to the rapid development of neighborhood health centers to serve the poor in medically deprived areas more effectively. But now the odds are that substantial new money to speed this expansion will not be forthcoming. In this connection one should recall that the British Health Act of 1946 anticipated the establishment of a large number of local clinics as one key to improving and rationalizing medical care. Yet it is only now—after twenty years —that the British have found a limited amount of resources for this purpose. Plans are one thing; execution another.

What do we know about the organizational structure of hospitals? First, some hospitals belong to the government. Most others are called "voluntary nonprofit," and a small percentage are proprietary institutions.

Since the federal government committed itself to increased funding of health services via Medicare and Medicaid, many businessmen have begun to respond by entering the field of nursing home operations. Nursing or convalescent homes appear to be potentially good business—witness the moves of Holiday Inn and other organizations in this direction. One consequence of such a development will be the introduction of modern management into the health services industry.

What can be said about the personnel practices of hospitals? Historically, the hospital was closely associated with the church. Its roots are deep in charity and good works. As a consequence it developed the stance that it was unnecessary to pay the staff a living wage. Traditionally people working in hospitals weren't expected to earn a living wage, and they didn't. As late as World War II leaders in Washington and elsewhere were outraged when nurses began to argue that they ought to be paid decently. This was demoralization. Nurses were ethically bound to work for the love of humanity. But such is no longer the case.

From almost every point of view, the hospital is an institutional anomaly. It is not yet fully acclimated to the modern world. It has taken the hospital more than twenty years to move from a quasi-protected environment rooted in philanthropy to a market economy. Who runs the hospital? One answer is that *nobody does.* The trustees don't; the hospital director cannot tell doctors what to do; the doctors disdain administration; the nurses are too preoccupied with jurisdictional squabbles. The answer nobody runs the hospital may help to account for the steeply rising costs.

Money and Manpower

For a great many generations, hospitals made a practice of getting on with very little money, using free labor as a substitute. This meant that they were little interested or concerned about paying competitive wages and in creating a sound personnel system responsive to the career needs of an increasingly differential work force. An employee with thirty years' service might earn the same as, or only a little more than, one with comparable skill who was hired last week.

Of late the situation has been further complicated by the fact that as more groups of specialists were hired—and many did not have true professional status—they nevertheless sought to mimic the exclusionary guild practices of the representative model—the physician. This meant that they sought to build a protective wall around themselves, making it that much harder to establish a career ladder for those who began at or close to the bottom.

No institution, no matter how deep its roots in tradition, can withstand the battering of reality. The charitable ethos of the hospital began to give way rapidly under the hard facts of new sources of funds from insurance and new shortages of manpower with the advent of a high-employment economy.

Third-party money has become ever more important. We still talk about "voluntary" hospitals, but one might ask, "What is 'voluntary' about a voluntary hospital?" Philanthropy contributes no more than 2.5 percent of the operating income of all general hospitals. Despite this small financial stake, philanthropy nonetheless continues to control the voluntary hospitals of the United States. This is less equity than is usually required for the effective control of a large corporation.

Actually, the bulk of the money used for hospitals today is third-party money, that is, money from insurance and government. At some point during this continuing financial transformation, hospital workers began to understand the shift in the source of operating funds and saw little or no point in agreeing to perpetuate a noncompetitive wage and salary structure to help cover the deficit. Professors at private universities still have to awaken to the fact that through their lower salaries they are helping to cover the deficit of the medical schools whose graduates will earn before too long between $35,000 and $50,000 annually.

Hospital workers finally decided that they had subsidized patients long enough; now third-party money could take over. The workers began to press their demands, but with each success new problems emerged. One fundamental argument was who should pay for the training of physicians, nurses, and other medical personnel, long an intrinsic hospital function. Third parties questioned whether it was their responsibility. They argued "We are not in the business of medical training; we are in the business of buying medical services." Whatever the merit of this position, it has helped to clarify the fact that the training of a physician in a hospital should not be assessed against a sweeper who earns $1.25 an hour. To complicate matters, nursing education has long been centered in the hospital. In the past, nursing education was an economic undertaking for the hospital, which received three years of nursing service from the student nurse in exchange for room, board, and minimum instruction. But times have changed, and most hospitals now lose money on nurses' training.

There are several avenues of possible adjustment. We must develop a more appropriate structure for nurses' education. There has recently been established one more commission under the chairmanship of Allen Wallis of Rochester University. It is hoped that this study will mark the end, at least for a time, of investigations of nursing education. But if it is to accomplish this, it will have to suggest how to free the hospital of the mounting costs of nurses' education and clarify who is to do the job of instruction and who is to pay for it.

Interns and residents, too, are pressing for a new deal, now that hospitals are making money for their services. Under the new reimbursement plans for Medicaid and Medicare, many hospitals earn substantial fees from the work of interns and residents. There is evidence from New York City and elsewhere that, with residents beginning to be paid $10,000 and more per year, a new division of the spoils will have to be made.

The Emergence of Collective Bargaining

It has taken but one generation, from the end of World War II to the recent past, for the hospital scene to be transformed from one where employees were expected to work for love and a little money to one where a recently organized union has succeeded in writing a contract which guarantees every worker, no matter how lowly his job, at least $100 a week. How can we explain so radical a change in so short a time?

Part of the explanation has already been suggested. The hospital became big business. It could grow only by attracting and holding an increasing proportion of the total labor force. Moreover, substantial new sources of reliable income have become available to hospitals which has greatly improved their position to hold their own in the scramble for scarce resources.

But there is more to the story. We must remember that the National Labor Relations Act exempted, after Taft-Hartley in 1947, hospitals and other nonprofit institutions from the necessity of dealing with unions. Further, all levels of government—federal, state, and local—looked with a jaundiced eye upon their employees' joining trade unions. We have, then, a sector of the economy, outnumbered in size only by agriculture and construction, in a special category with regard to its labor relations. But recently both law and administrative practice have begun to change in a way that permits hospital workers to organize.

In the early 1960s, following the lead of New York City, the federal government made it possible for its civil service employees, including specifically hospital workers, to join unions of their choosing. And various progressive states soon followed in its path. Of course permission was granted for workers to organize and join unions, not to go out on strike. But this prohibition has been repeatedly breached. Similarly, changes in federal and state laws and administrative practices have lifted the prior exemption of many nonprofit organizations, including hospitals, from having to negotiate with unions.

The fact that various health professionals and workers

have on occasion engaged in extreme behavior—walking off the job or refusing to come to work, in short, striking in fact if not always in name—has driven the lesson home that hospitals are no longer immune from the consequences of failure in collective bargaining that have long been part of the experience of the private sector.

The changes noted above do not mean that most hospitals in the United States have been unionized or are likely to become so in the near future. What has actually happened so far is a beginning change in the labor relations climate from one totally hostile to unionization to one which brings organization and collective bargaining within the realm of possibility.

Trade unions are like other large organizations—universities, the federal government, corporations. They are usually top-heavy, inept, and slow to respond to change. This helps to explain why they have moved slowly into the field of medical services. But they have begun to move. They have recognized, even though belatedly, that the time is ripe. They hesitated to move earlier because of the antagonism of the public. Unions did not underestimate the dangers of pulling workers out of a hospital to enforce their demands but, without resort to striking, they had little prospect of getting their demands accepted.

The American Nurses Association decided in 1946 that continuing to be ladylike was no longer an effective posture and therefore authorized its constituent state associations to bargain for their members. It appears that these efforts have been productive in about 10 percent of the cases undertaken and have had some slight influence in another 15 percent. This suggests that nurses may still be too ladylike. They occasionally threaten to strike; they seldom do.

In many cities, the local Hospital Association is well organized. Until faced with acute manpower shortages, the members operated in consort in labor matters. However, when the market became very tight, the workers were in a more favorable position to bargain. The unions were also faced with vigorously resistant hospital boards. The trustees of voluntary hospitals, businessmen who had seen their department stores, their factories, and their trucking fleets organized, decided to make a last stand. If a man couldn't beat the union in the private economy, he could at least stand up to it in discharging his public responsibilities. After all, it was the trustees' duty to protect the patient.

The present is always intermediary between the past and the future. It would appear on the basis of a preliminary analysis that while unionization has made some headway recently, it is not making rapid progress and there is little prospect that it will in the near or even more distant future. But such a conclusion would be justified only if the underlying factors influencing the bargaining position of workers and management in the health services industry were operating to support the status quo. Let us briefly review the evidence.

The American economy is being transformed as the labor force shifts increasingly from the production of goods to the provision of services. Clearly a trade-union movement based initially in manufacturing does not have a rosy future unless it shifts its attention increasingly toward the service sector and seeks new members there. The unions have no option but to organize service workers.

A second related transformation is the growth of the not-for-profit sector. Today close to 2 out of 5 workers are employed on government account and by nonprofit institutions. Once again the unions have little option but to pay particular attention to this rapidly growing sector.

Here then are two principal factors—the trend toward services and the trend toward the not-for-profit sector—that foreshadow more and more union preoccupation with the organization of hospital workers. And there are additional trends operating in the economy and the society that reinforce these pressures. There is the matter of urbanization. More and more we are becoming a people who live in metropolitan centers and, other things being equal, the more concentrated the population, the easier it is to interest them in joining a union. Then there is the matter of the size of the hospital. Increasingly the large medical institution is the prototype and size is likewise conducive to organization.

But the most interesting dimension—and the one that is likely to contribute most to unionization—is the fact that in a majority of our large cities a high proportion of the less-skilled members of the hospital work force are members of minority groups, primarily Negroes. We find here an intersection between the racial revolution and the thrust toward unionization. As the experience of Local 1199 in New York City has demonstrated, under effective leadership, the frustrations of minorities can serve as a potent stimulus to organizing the lowly paid and the unskilled.

The fact that an increasing proportion of all hospital income comes from government and from quasi-commercial organizations, such as Blue Cross, points up the importance of the growth of political power and influence of minority groups. The ability of a union to organize hospital workers will often depend on whether or not the union leadership can gain the support, or at least the neutrality, of the Mayor and his aides. This interplay between unionization and the growth of local political power for minority groups can be read in recent developments on both the East and the West Coasts. Those who believe that unions have little future in the hospital field had better test the hypothesis that minority groups are likely to gain political power, particularly at the level of local government. For if the latter occurs, the former is not likely to obtain.

Three statements in conclusion. The personnel practices of most hospitals are anachronistic for a $55 billion health services industry. They reek of paternalism, protectionism, and exploitation. They have long been predicated on hiring the largest number at the lowest wage and ignoring to a large extent the relations between incentives and productivity.

Second, trade-union organization, if it is effective, can make a contribution to improving manpower utilization in hospitals by insisting that the price of labor be adjusted to the competitive market. This will force hospital administrators to devote more time and effort to using their labor efficiently.

Third, we may soon be confronted in the United States with the need to develop an incomes policy. Firemen want more money, bus drivers want more money, sanitation workers want more money, hospital workers want more money. With 2 out of 5 people working in the not-for-profit sector, the question of a substitute for the competitive market in setting wages cannot be skirted indefinitely. An answer must be found, but it will not come quickly.

❧ 5 ❧
What Price Medicaid?

Although several years have passed since Congress enacted Medicaid as a companion measure to Medicare, few people would be able to describe it with any precision. The new Medical Assistance Program is not a single program but potentially fifty-four separate ones, based on the principle of federal cost-sharing with the states at a rate varying from 50 to 83 percent, depending on the level at which the states are able to provide medical care for welfare recipients and the medically indigent.

The federal legislation established the minimum services that must be provided: each state program must cover all recipients under the welfare categories to which the federal government contributes and must make available to them at least five basic services—inpatient and outpatient hospital care, physicians' services, X-ray and laboratory services, and skilled nursing-home care. But states could go far beyond this minimum and include in the plans people who are self-supporting except for medical expenditures, the "medically indigent." They could also add other services to the minimum five.

A large majority—36 states, the District of Columbia, Puerto Rico, and the Virgin Islands—have risen to the federal bait. But, as of 1967, Guam and 14 states, including most of the South and such preserves of the status quo as New Jersey, Indiana, and Colorado, were still outside the system. This reflects their unwillingness or inability to provide even the required 17 percent or more of the funds. Most of these states do not provide sufficient funds to enable their poor to receive even state-approved minimum allowances for food and other essentials. It is likely, however, that the recalcitrants will join before 1970, since under the terms of the law they would otherwise forfeit medical care reimbursement on behalf of welfare recipients already receiving federal help: the blind, families with dependent children, the aged, and the disabled.

Of the 39 jurisdictions that had established a Medicaid program by the fall of 1967, 15 have restricted their plans to welfare recipients while 24 include the medically indigent. Only Wyoming limits itself to the federally established minimum services; the rest provide from one to twenty additional services. A few states provide for more services to welfare recipients than to the medically indigent. The variability among states even with respect to the basic five services is substantial. Montana allows only a total of 14 days of inpatient care per year, while Idaho allows 20 days for each admission. In Louisiana a patient may visit a doctor twice in one month; in Utah patients with chronic illnesses are limited to one visit per month. When drugs are covered, they usually have a $10-to-$15 monthly ceiling or are allowed only for inpatients. But the most important difference among the various state plans lies in the wide spread among the annual income levels used to determine medical indigence—a high of $2,900 for a single adult and $6,000 for a family of four in New York, and a corresponding low of $1,728 and $2,448 in Oklahoma.[1]

In its second session, the Ninetieth Congress reacted to New York's combination of high eligibility limits and virtually open-ended benefits and their implications for federal reimbursement levels by amending the Medicaid legislation to define as medical indigents persons whose income did not exceed welfare subsistence levels by more than 33 percent. Congress was led to act by the realization that under the New York plan about a third of the state's population was eligible for Medicaid, although a much smaller proportion had actually registered (it had been anticipated that by the end of 1968 about half of the eligibles would be enrolled). Since the *average* annual individual bill for services in 1967-68 was about $450, the potential liability of the federal government for Medicaid in New York State alone could amount to 6 million persons times $225, or $1.35 billion annually. This figure, moreover, is based on the premise that medical services will not rise in cost, an assumption at variance with recent experience.[2]

The congressional restrictions brought angry protests from the New York State delegation, from Governor Rockefeller, and from Mayor John V. Lindsay of New York City, all of whom reasonably resent the imbalance between taxes paid by their state and moneys received from the federal treasury. But Medicaid is hardly the appropriate instrument for rectifying this fundamental fiscal anomaly. The amount of New York's claims for federal reimbursement for Medicaid was close to the figure initially estimated for the entire country. Unless Medicaid was to become a form of federal encouragement to the prosperous and progressive states, Congress had no option but to stop and reconsider the road that it had begun to travel.

It has been argued for years that the United States was lagging far behind most Western European countries by failing to include health, at least for the poor, among the services for which government accepts responsibility. Despite their victory with Medicare, proponents of social reform recognized that old people represent only a minority of all those whose health needs would remain unmet without expanded federal responsibility. Medicare–Medicaid was seen as a major extension of the 1960 Kerr–Mills Social Security Amendment, which had sought, through the lure of federal dollars, to stimulate the development of state programs for providing health services to medically indigent persons above the age of 65. It is difficult to blame Congress for voting in 1965 to include health within an expanded welfare program; clearly it was responding to a long-felt need. If criticism is justified, it might be directed to the legislators' disregard of the complications, their underestimation of the sums that would be involved, and their overoptimism concerning the ease of providing better medical care for all of those unable to pay.

It is difficult to imagine that Congress believed it could effect a radical transformation in the medical situation of low-income families simply by the injection of between $1 billion to $2 billion into a total annual national health bill of around $55 billion. Even after matching funds by states are added, this is a modest increment to the total. The legislators, then, were taking what seemed to them one modest step forward.

It is more difficult to interpret what advocates of the legislation had in mind. Even though they are unrelenting opponents of a means test and probably had few illusions that Medicaid could bring a high level of medical care to the poor and near-poor, they must have felt that it would serve as a basis for more far-reaching improvements.

With the legislators willing and the proponents of medical reform satisfied that they had nothing to lose, indirect help appeared in the form of relative complaisance from an unlikely quarter—the AMA. Shaken by the defeat they had suffered in the long fight over Medicare, the leaders of organized medicine had neither the resources nor the inclination to battle against Medicaid. Moreover, they have always been relatively relaxed about policies and programs aimed at providing services for the poor, who are of minor consequence in private practice. Since Medicaid had been drafted to assure free choice of physician, fee for service, freedom for the physician to join the system, and most of the other safeguards demanded by the AMA, why should the leadership put up more than a token fight? The impact of the new legislation would be to turn charity cases into paying patients.

Hospitals looked forward eagerly to having their bills paid. Governors and mayors especially from the more progressive states saw the prospect that their health and welfare budgets would be eased by an infusion of new federal money.

With hindsight, it is clear that any legislation that found favor among such disparate groups must have been radically awry from the outset. Everyone was to get something, yet give little or nothing in return. With Congress putting in very little additional money (so it thought), the advocates of medical reform saw the opportunity for a major move to reshape the prevailing system of providing medical services to people with low incomes, and all this without disturbing the entrepreneurial freedom of the medical profession to any significant degree.

The hospitals, at least, have not been disappointed. They have received the bulk of the moneys paid out by Medicaid. Moreover, under the "reasonable cost" provision, in many states they have been able to raise substantially the rates that they charge. Several hospitals in New York City charge more than $90 a day for Medicaid patients, about twice what they were paid by the state government less than two years ago.[3] Nor has this been the total extent of their gain. Since Medicaid pays for outpatient care, hospitals now claim reimbursement at the rate of $20 to $25 per outpatient visit. In some cases this represents a several hundredfold increase over previous state reimbursement rates.

The complaisance of the doctors has also been largely justified. Many participating physicians complain bitterly about the red tape that has delayed their payments, some are restive about the arbitrary manner in which their bills have been reduced, and others are concerned about the high eligibility limits in certain states for certification for medical indigency. But New York City's announcement in December, 1967, that thenceforth it would audit the bills of participating physicians whose requests for reimbursements exceed $5,000 monthly appears to bear out the AMA's perception that it could live with Medicaid.

What about the anticipation that Medicaid would lead the poor at least part of the way toward receiving the benefits of American medicine? The first point at issue is the definition of the poor. If New York's original income standards were followed and applied to the nation as a whole, close to half the population would be found medically indigent. There is no evidence that *quality* medical care carries a substantially different price tag in different parts of the country. The real reason for the wide discrepancy in the definition of medical indigency among the states reflects disparities in social attitudes, fiscal capacity, and medical standards.

In short, arithmetic stands in the way of delivering a reasonable level of medical care to all the people if we adopt as a norm the quantity and quality of care that the more prosperous states hope to provide. If Medicaid sought to bring the 30 million defined as poor by the Office of Economic Opportunity—about 15 percent of the population—into the established system, it would prove a difficult but potentially manageable task. But 50 percent is something else again. Even before the program was in full swing, Governor Ronald Reagan of California and Governor Nelson Rockefeller of New York sought cutbacks in their states' support for what is turning out to be an exceedingly expensive effort.

A second assumption that warrants closer inspection is

that the opening of a new source of financing for medical care while all other parts of the system are left substantially intact will provide the recipients with much better care than before. There is no denying that voluntary hospitals are now inclined to admit and treat patients who have been certified for Medicaid and that physicians who are participating in the program are willing to treat them. Money does count, and a poor man with new-found funds is better off. But money in the pockets of the poor is not suddenly transmuted into more doctors, more special services and facilities, and more approved nursing homes. Most medical resources were tight before Medicaid, and they have become tighter since. The poor and near poor must still compete with those who have more income, and it is optimistic indeed to expect private physicians to set up practice in the poverty areas of the Northern cities because many indigent Negroes are now certified for Medicaid. (Indeed, it is doubtful whether more than 15 percent of the physicians in New York City are regularly participating in any effective way in providing services under Medicaid.)[4] Finally, no one has yet demonstrated how the 14 million rural poor, 11 million of whom are white, according to the President's Commission on Rural Poverty, are suddenly or even slowly to obtain more and better medical services than in the past. A few billion dollars of additional financing can neither add significantly to the pool of medical resources nor do much to redistribute existing resources in favor of the poor.

What has happened and what will happen is reasonably clear. The purveyors of medical services will continue to benefit from the new infusion of funds; hospitals will have fewer bad debts; physicians will no longer adjust their bills downward or fail to collect; pharmacists will enjoy increased sales. All this was inevitable since the aim of the legislation was to disturb nothing in a system that medical planners have repeatedly indicted as unplanned, inefficient, wasteful, and exploitative. The best that could result from the infusion of modest additional federal funds was that the states would liberalize the terms under which they would provide medical services. The majority of states have responded, and persons certified for Medicaid have made some palpable gains, but it would be indulging in fantasy to believe that under the present law the poor will be treated to the best that American medicine has to offer.

No country in the world has been able to equalize the quantity and quality of medical services rendered the rich and poor, the urban dweller and the farmer. The Soviet Union and Great Britain have been able to establish a minimum level of services for all citizens only through a national system in which the government has substantial control over all medical resources, including physicians. Admittedly we are much richer than either of these countries. But this fact also makes it easier for many Americans to be reasonably satisfied with a system of medical care which may be expensive but to which they have access.

There is no possible way of defining a third to a half of our entire population as entitled to medical care at government expense without a revolutionary restructuring of American medicine that would include control over doctors. Until major changes are brought about in American life, the present highly imperfect system based on consumer dependence, physicians' freedom, community autonomy, and governmental impotence is apt to persist, even as its desultory transformation continues. Meanwhile, since politics is the art of accomplishing the possible, it would seem the better part of wisdom to concentrate on a limited number of objectives with a reasonable prospect of success, such as improving ambulatory services, nursing homes, and preventive medicine for children in the schools, and by ensuring that government funds are used more effectively for the poor.

PART TWO
The Medical
Profession

✌ 6 ✌
The Physician and Market Power

One cannot talk in the abstract about manpower. One can talk about manpower only in terms of institutional structures or the leverages of different groups to affect demand and supply.

Every few weeks, months, or years some group of leaders in the Congress or the administration decides that the United States is facing a crisis in medicine, medical manpower, and medical costs. And they call a hearing, a meeting, or a conference to deal with the emergency. Experts make speeches, the speeches are discussed, proceedings are published, and the crisis is resolved until the next time.

The question that is worth raising is what lies back of this recurrent crisis in American medicine? The answer seems to lie in the sudden wide gap that has been introduced between our expectations and our abilities to meet them. It has been stated authoritatively that everybody has a right to quality medical care, provided as a personalized service, in a dignified way, without a waste of time and without jeopardizing his personal budget. But this is nonsense. We have never had such a system in this country, except possibly for the professors of surgery who have their families treated by the professors of medicine. Even that is questionable, since even professors at major institutions who earn good salaries and who are friendly with members of the medical faculty frequently get poor medical care. It has little to do with lack of funds; it has little to do with lack of education. Yet it seems to be true. A truly satisfactory system of medical care never existed for more than a few of the wealthy. It was slowly expanded to encompass a proportion of the affluent middle class. Certainly we never had an adequate system for the average citizen or for the poor.

We cannot suddenly redefine the goals of a system that has been satisfying perhaps a quarter of the population to include quality care for the entire population without runing into difficulties that quickly become reflected in shortages of funds, facilities, and staff.

Under the doctrine of a brave new world for all, we will continue to have manpower shortages of every type. There are not enough doctors or nurses or other types of medical manpower at the moment to fulfill this commitment. Therefore additional doctors, nurses, and technicians will be produced. However, discrepancies will continue to exist between the services that have been promised and the people available to provide them. Therefore more staff will be sought. We now have 3 to 4 million people in the health industry. And unless the idealistic goals just outlined are modified, manpower shortages will persist.

The explanation must be sought in an anomaly of the medical market. In most markets, supply and demand are kept in reasonable balance through the movements of prices. But since the nation has declared that people are entitled to quality medical care irrespective of their ability to pay for it, and since affluent consumers are prepared to put their extra income into the purchase of services, including medical services—from orthodontia to psychoanalysis—the adjustment mechanism operates differently. The control on expansion is not the price mechanism but is determined primarily by the availability of the supply. In short, the supply of medical resources has thus far effectively generated its own demand!

A further interesting insight into the medical market is provided by the AMA's recent reversal of policy which led it to favor the expansion of the supply of physicians. This is understandable only if the AMA believes that Congress and the public will be willing to continue spending enormous sums of money for medical services. Under these circumstances, the AMA is interested in increasing the number of physicians. Once the leadership has become convinced that the U.S. Treasury is back of the medical system, and once the principle of fee-for-service has been accepted, with the doctor determining how much service is needed, then it is indeed utopia . . . for the physician.

The AMA saw no contradiction in favoring a rapid expansion in the supply of physicians at the same time that it warned against the steep rise in medical costs. Yet experts such as Professor Rashi Fein have warned that one of the ways most certain to bring about further rapid rises in medical costs is to attempt to solve the shortages of medical manpower by training more physicians. Although the

AMA might prefer it, we cannot have it both ways. We cannot be interested in securing a more rational use of human resources with an aim of better accomplishing certain specific ends and simultaneously decide that the best answer to existing shortages is to continue the pattern that has resulted in the present gap between our resources and our goals.

In the United States we have talked for years about how medical care should be reorganized to make it more effective, more efficient, better in every way. The discussions go on, but little happens because those who want the changes have no market power to bring them about. And those who have the market power are not interested in changes. The members of the key professions that provide medical care are generally satisfied with the existing structure. We are not a police state. This means that each profession determines the way it practices. Each profession is willing to have conferences periodically to discuss broad issues. However, nothing is likely to change if the leadership is satisfied with the status quo.

Discussion about regionalization started in the late 1930s. However, physicians do not want to transfer patients to other physicians, because they make their living from patients. That is a fact. That is why little was done to implement regionalization plans. The Rochester plan and that of Bingham Associates, among others, did not work out well. Their success was limited in area and in time. The plans did not demonstrate that regionalization incorporated a capacity for growth with better coordination and integration. Moreover, the experiments in the East were not copied in other areas of the country. The effort was still-born.

Much the same conclusion can be drawn about group practice, especially group practice of the variety that medical reform has for so long assumed holds the key to a vast improvement in the entire system—prepaid comprehensive group medicine in which both ambulatory and inpatient services are provided. Here the record is slightly better but only slightly. The few plans, such as Kaiser Permanente, that have proved satisfactory had some special circumstances such as a major assist from a corporate or governmental employer.[1]

Admittedly these plans had to fight an uphill battle against the medical establishment, but it is too easy to put all or even most of the blame for their slow growth onto the backs of the AMA leadership. More likely both physicians and patients have had their doubts about this approach.

It is odd that after incorporating the U.S. Treasury into the medical system, Congressman Wilbur Mills has stated that he is worried about a crisis! His crisis is a congressional crisis about money. With more money flowing in, it will be harder to effect a reorganization in medicine. Why should a system change if there is an abundance of money? The elementary principle in all organizations is that they change only under dire threats to their survival. Institutions that have no serious problems do not change. As far as practicing physicians and hospitals are concerned, they are being reimbursed liberally and they feel no pressure to change.

The U.S. government pays for education and training at different levels in the medical arena without asking any return from the various professional groups. It is no secret that it is hard to induce young physicians with college-educated wives to live in rural areas. This is true in every country, including Russia. With a predominant number of women physicians, Russia has faced particular difficulties in physician allocation.

It is perfectly proper for a democracy to ask a return for financial assistance. If we agree to subsidize medical education or any other kind of education, there is no reason not to require a few years of service in places to which it is difficult to attract trained persons. We could say to a young man, "We will put you through a residency but then you will owe the government a certain number of years of service." If the problem of rural coverage is serious, a solution can be found. It is a question of whether the democracy really wants to find a solution.

Usually, the organization of medical services outside the hospital is a function of what suits the bulk of the practitioners. They determine it. Practitioners decide who gives services to whom, and who gets charged for what. Clearly, the long-term pattern of provision of medical services outside of hospitals has been satisfactory to most practitioners.

Several years ago I asked my ophthalmologist, a brilliant physician and surgeon, why he continued to do refractions. "What can be more boring for you than to sit hour after hour and do refractions? Why don't you let your nurse do it? Or your assistant?" He replied, "Don't be naive. You pay me $25 or $35 to refract your eyes. If my assistant or the nurse did it, how could I get that fee?" It was as simple as that.

Obviously, the American consumer cannot be reeducated overnight. It will take time and effort to wean the consumer away from sole reliance on the physician and to gain his consent to have allied health personnel take over many duties now performed by the physician. The medical profession, which earns its livelihood by practicing, finds the present system satisfactory. The consumer doesn't seem to object to it. We are told that there is a big crisis in medical care, but consumer lethargy leads one to question whether a crisis does in fact exist.

There will never be a significant readjustment of American medical practice until the physician takes a major role in reeducating the patient. The doctor must say, "The nurse is going to examine your eyes." Or, "The ophthalmologic assistant has more patience and will do it better than I will. I will make sure there is no pathologic disease before you leave." Now, that is the only way the American public can be reeducated. But why should the physician be interested in reeducating the patients who support him in fine style?

The hospital is a unique social institution. A hospital takes community capital and structures a workplace for the physician and a treatment place for the patient. A large part of hospital development is for the convenience and effectiveness of the practicing physician. It is a great help to the physician to have all of his patients collected under one roof. It is such a help that a few doctors submitted bills to Medicaid amounting to $16,000 for four months work because their patients were located in one place and they were able to see 25 patients per hour![2]

These are extreme cases of exploitation of patients, the community, and the government. But the fact remains that the American people have never looked carefully at the large investments in hospital plant and operations they underwrite or the extent of the costs that ensue because the hospital is operated for the convenience of the physician. What other explanation is there for the fact that all surgery, except emergencies, is performed during the first five days of the week and usually only in the morning?

The present concept of a hospital administrator is largely a contradiction in terms. He doesn't manage anybody except possibly housekeeping personnel. No hospital administrator dares make suggestions to the chief of surgery, the chief of medicine, or to the chief nurse, if he wants to keep his job. He formally directs all these resources, but he does not control them. And, therefore, he cannot change anything—at least not anything important!

All this is a simple way to emphasize that if one wants to talk about manpower utilization, one must talk about power. Market power is necessary to change resource inputs and their patterns of utilization. In our society, that kind of power does not exist anywhere in today's hospital.

It is interesting to note the areas in which the AMA has been relaxed about radical changes in medical practice. Historically, the AMA never worried about medical services to the poor. Their medical services could be provided in almost any way; there could be a closed hospital group running good clinics or bad clinics, but the poor were never the preoccupation of organized medicine. Experimentation and innovation with services for the poor were possible because the poor did not affect the central stream of purchasing power. In the past, most medical reforms related to the poor—and this continues today. For instance, the Office of Economic Opportunity (OEO) today has some interesting community health experiments under way. The OEO was able to start these before opposition was mobilized against them. When physicians have more than enough paying patients to take all of their time, and innovations do not threaten to become generalized, they do not worry about a group of social reformers restructuring medical services for the poor.

That is how medical services for the poor were started, but that is not how they will end. Medicare and Medicaid changed the financial status of the poor—at least with regard to medical services. No longer do they have to ask charity of the physician or the hospital or seek to persuade the welfare commissioner that they require care. Government has made them "financially responsible." The AMA was not slow to catch on. It has begun to raise questions about the propriety of structuring the community health centers along the lines that the OEO has been willing to approve.

There is a further aspect to the economic transformation of the poor with regard to medical services that may yet lead to radical changes in the basic structure of medical education and hospital care. Until now it was the poor who provided the teaching material on which the young physician practiced and learned. But with the poor now able to pay for medical care with government moneys, the old pattern is certain to be disrupted. The outlines of the new are just taking shape. Here is further proof that significant changes are dependent on market power and that market power is a function of control over money.

Most of this discussion about market power has been focused on the physician, since he is at the apex of the system of medical care. However, all the other allied health professionals seek to do exactly the same as physicians, within the limits of their power. For instance, over the years registered nurses have done their utmost to keep practical nurses and nurse's aides from usurping any of their power or influence. They have fought hard and long to protect their domain and keep the new groups from getting a piece of the action. Each of the other large groups in the medical care industry follows the same general approach of seeking to protect its domain and enlarge its market power.

Now, if there is no medical crisis, what should be done? One preference is to be cautious about intervening in the system. It is not a perfect system by any means, and its critics have little difficulty in drawing up a long list of indictments against it. Yet the system has been able to contribute to a modest prolongation of life and to a substantial reduction of pain and discomfort.

It is by now anachronistic and perhaps not even politically safe to raise questions about the wisdom of Medicare, but there are a few "mossheads" who still inquire whether the country did not pay too much for Medicare when it got Medicaid in the bargain. The purchase price included a system of "fee-for-service" and hospital reimbursement on a "cost plus" basis. It still remains to be proved that even the richest country in the world can live with a system that gives the purveyors of services direct access to the U.S. Treasury!

If we have no crisis and if there is something to be said for not seeking to alter everything at once—which cannot be done anyhow because those who hold market power are not interested in radical changes—what should be the direction of reform? Presumably some reforms are desirable.

Some contend that past trends should be continued and that it is sound to broaden the education and training of all members of the medical profession, particularly that of physicians and nurses. They see the strength of the system in well-trained practitioners and specialists. And there is much to be said in favor of training in depth. Yet the recent Carnegie–Commonwealth Conference on Medical Education heard a distinguished surgeon from Harvard say that he never understood why certain specialty boards permitted one to become a specialist and operate on certain organs of the body after two years, while other specialty boards required five years of residency before one was permitted to operate on other organs.[3] We ought to make more sense than this out of the relationship between the years of education and training and later performance.

It should be clear, however, that we cannot indefinitely extend the period of training on the assumption that the more the better. In this connection it is well to recall Dr. Lewin's study of some years ago which disclosed the amazing fact that an average fully fledged member of the American Psychoanalytic Association did not complete all of his training until after his fortieth year. Small wonder that psychoanalysts charge large fees. They have only a short time in which to recover for years of outlay.

There are many hospital administrators and physicians who are unsettled by what has been transpiring in the field of nursing. The leadership of the American Nurses Association has advocated that more nurses complete a baccalaureate degree before entering upon their profession. But those who have the responsibility for staffing institutions and for seeing that patients are looked after question whether this recommendation is not misplaced, since most functions that nurses perform, especially within the supervised environment of the hospital, can be learned within a period of weeks, surely months, rather than years.

There is a tremendous tendency in America to add years of education without making the training functional to needs. We used to be able to go through public school and learn how to read, write, and do arithmetic. Then high school and college were added for the average American. Yet many students still do not control the fundamentals. It makes no sense that any system, medical or other, should simply strive to elongate indefinitely the educational–training process. A first effort of reform should be to control and cut back on any unnecessary extension of the training process. It is costly to the individual and wasteful from the viewpoint of society.

A second direction for reform points at that expensive institution, the hospital. We must get management into that institution and secure power for its administrative head.

Boards of trustees have been reprehensible because they have the legal power—they, not the physicians. However, some physicians who treat the trustees might be in a position to determine how this power is used. In the military, medical departments have always had a considerable degree of autonomy, a considerable degree of power, because it is their responsibility to determine whether an officer should be retired for reasons of health. This gives the medical officer a trump card. The physician who treats trustees also holds some good trumps. Obviously, if a hospital is going to be reorganized sensibly, power has to be in the hands of those who are to run it. Without power nothing will be changed. If we want to control costs and manpower utilization, the first and most important aim should be to get the hospital under control. A rational, efficient, centralized administrative approach does not now exist. It can come into being only if the director or administrator is given the power to make important decisions over clinical services.

A third recommendation reflects the fact that the medical industry, broadly defined, employs over 3 million people. More than a million are professionals with at least a baccalaureate degree. However, the difficulty that confronts the industry is that it employs many women. Women are not as career-oriented as men. Women are a relatively cheap labor resource. One reason that we have not improved our manpower utilization in the health industry is its predominantly female labor force. The industry should take steps to attract more men; it should develop better career-progression lines.

Any significant program to improve manpower utilization within the hospital, as well as outside, carries with it
a new division of the medical dollar. At present, there is a
wide gap between the earnings of the physician and those
of the people who help him. It is questionable whether a
realistic study of the contribution of allied health personnel to the total system would justify the present pattern of
income distribution. Yet it will not be easy to obtain agreement from the medical profession about a new division.
The best prospect of making a change is within the hospital, where the lay board of trustees might be convinced to
take the lead in helping to bring that about as one part of
a larger plan to rationalize the use of manpower resources.

Americans are medicine-mad. The public doesn't understand that most illnesses are self-limiting. It doesn't understand that for most chronic illnesses the physician can
do little. That is what is meant by chronicity. The public
has a simple view about the cutting edge of medicine. Obviously, if one is in a serious accident, quick admission to
a hospital may be of critical importance. But emergency
situations account for a relatively small part of medicine.

There are at least two other kinds of intervention. One
may be neutral but costly. Another kind of medical intervention may be costly and negative. It is no secret to the
insiders that the amount of unnecessary surgery in certain
fields runs between 25 to 50 percent. The American public
does not have a realistic view of the nature of American
medicine. Medicine is lifesaving and can be tremendously
important at the margin. With respect to most run-of-the-
mill conditions, however, it is palliative, it is supportive.

This does not minimize the importance that patients attach to their ability to turn over their medical problems to an expert. It is—and should be—a source of comfort, even if the intervention of the expert has little effect on the outcome.

The younger age groups in America have, on the average, thirteen years of formal education. There must be some way of changing the system of medical services in this country to take cognizance of the fact that we have a constantly better educated public. Otherwise we fail to profit from the dynamic progress that our society is making. Modern medicine is an outgrowth of a highly authoritarian system in which the physician stood on high and the poor ignorant patient belonged to a lower species. But since more and more of our population graduates from high school and college, the time has surely come to look anew at the role of the individual in maintaining his own health, in seeking medical attention, and in following the regimen that the physician prescribes. The effectiveness of a medical system surely depends on the quality of the professionals who provide the services. But whether they will be able to provide the required services in time and whether the services they provide will be effective will in large measure depend on the insight and cooperation of the patient. We may be able to cut considerably our requirements for professional manpower if we devote a little more time and effort to the physician of first resort—the citizen. Crisis or no, a more effective system of medical care requires that the citizen play a larger role in the preservation of his health.

～7～

The Physician Shortage
Reconsidered

It is never popular to argue against the trend, especially when all the "good" people are on one side. Nevertheless, once in a while a skeptic can make his voice heard above the prevailing wind. For at least the last decade all the good people have known that the United States needs more physicians and that only the reactionary leadership of the AMA has prevented the launching of adequate programs to increase the supply. The distinguished *New England Journal of Medicine* noted in its December 3, 1959 issue that an economist had raised some questions before a congressional committee about the need for more physicians, and in its February 18, 1960 issue it published a further comment on the subject.

Now, six years later, and with the Bayne–Jones and Bain reports, the National Institutes of Health Report on Manpower for Medical Research, the Recommendations of the Sub-Committee on Manpower of the Commission on Heart Disease, Cancer and Stroke, the *Health Manpower Source Book* (Section 18), and more recently the report of the President's Advisory Commission on Health Manpower

(1967) as reference sources, let us reconsider this question.[1]

A week-long conference on medical education in 1966, attended by leaders in the field and a few outsiders, concluded that it was not only desirable but essential that the supply of physicians be increased by at least 4 percent per annum over the next decade or so. What does an increase of 4 percent per annum mean?[2]

From an annual output of about 8,000 the number of graduates should increase to 12,000 a decade hence. The Ft. Lauderdale Conference was reacting to the government forecast which showed an annual output of only slightly more than 9,000 for 1975. When allowance is made for the graduates of Canadian and foreign medical schools, the government's estimate contemplated a modest increase in the ratio of physicians per 100,000 population—from 150 to 154. But the conferees were not satisfied with so small a gain. They recommended action that would increase the graduating class in 1975 to a level of about 30 percent above the government's forecast. What lay back of this proposal for such a radical increase?

The principal reasons that were adduced encompassed: the rate of population increase, the loss of physicians by retirement or death, the increased demand for physicians' services resulting from higher consumer income and new governmental programs such as Medicare, and the increasing time that physicians must spend with patients as a result of new medical and surgical procedures.

The foregoing stresses the important quantitative parameters that were likely to necessitate an increased supply of physicians. But the conferees were also much interested in how an enlarged supply could contribute to important qualitative gains in the provision of medical services. They called attention to the desirability of adding to the output so as to improve the mix between the younger, better trained men and the older practitioners who were often out of touch with recent developments. Moreover they saw no escape from the dependence of many hospitals for house staff on poorly trained foreign physicians except by a substantial addition to the output of American graduates. They further stipulated that only a loosening of the tautness in the domestic supply would encourage the service overseas of more American physicians, something that the Conference viewed with favor. They believed that the United States could gain much good will and contribute significantly to the welfare of the developing nations through greater participation on the medical front.

Along parallel lines, they saw little prospect of improving the medical services received by the disadvantaged at home unless the number of physicians was substantially increased. And finally it was their considered opinion that American physicians worked too long and too hard, but they saw little likelihood of reducing the pressure on them except through a substantially enlarged supply.

How can a reasonable man be unpersuaded by such weighty claims? Yet here are some of the reasons that at least one participant continued to voice his skepticism, not about the desirability of increasing the supply of physicians, but at defining the situation as a crisis and calling for a forced increase of large magnitude.

The Conference assumed that our population is increasing at the rate of 2 percent per annum. In point of fact, the current rate of increase is below 1.2 percent.[3] To postulate a 2 percent rate of increase means an error of more than 50 percent in the demand predicated on this crucial factor.

Rising income is not new. The per capita income of the United States has increased about threefold since the turn of this century, while the physician–population ratio actually declined between 1900 and 1960. Clearly, real per capita income and the number of physicians do not have to increase in tandem unless one wants to argue that there has been a decline in the quantity and quality of medical care available to the American people during this century—a position that the conferees would of course not support. Medicare will certainly lead to a small increased demand for physicians' services, but its greatest impact is likely to be on the demand for additional nursing services.[4]

Again, it is reasonable to stress that certain new medical and surgical procedures will require a large amount of physicians' time, but it is hard to believe, as some contended, that all the "slack" in the utilization of physicians' time has been squeezed out of the system. One participant called attention to a report which shows that 50 percent of a pediatrician's time in his office is devoted to procedures that paramedical personnel can equally well perform. Clearly, one must still look for gains in productivity.[5]

One can accept the conclusion that physicians trained after World War II are better prepared than the older members of the profession—a conclusion that was forcefully advanced. However, the overwhelming proportion of all physicians in active practice in 1975 will belong to this group.

Some foreign-trained physicians are Americans. But the majority are foreigners who cannot return home or who do not want to after completing their advanced training here. An arbitrary refusal to license them would simply force many to move to another country. This does not imply that the rich United States should continue to recruit physicians abroad, nor even that it should continue without change its immigration and employment policies that act to attract physicians from abroad.

Some time ago President Johnson announced a program to expand the role of the United States in helping to raise the health standards of developing nations. But experience has demonstrated that the numbers of physicians likely to be involved will not be large. More than physicians, Asia and Africa need sanitarians, veterinarians, and public health nurses.

It can be stipulated that our disadvantaged populations in rural and urban areas need more and better health services, but the critical question is whether the graduation annually of an additional 1,000 physicians in the Northeast would in fact assure such services either for the slum population of New York City or for poor whites and Negroes in the rural areas of Mississippi. Moreover, although the poor undoubtedly need better medical care, it is not irrelevant to inquire where this stands in the priority of their needs. It might make more sense for a concerned society to see to it that many of the poor first have the opportunity to work, to earn a decent income, to support their families.

Everyone knows that many physicians work too many hours and far too many years. But this is not simply because there is no one to take their place. Most independent professionals work hard because they want to. Moreover, most independent professionals work beyond their sixty-fifth year because they want to. It is the practitioner working alone in a rural area who is likely to keep going until he drops in his tracks. But increasing the annual number of graduates is not likely to provide him with a replacement.

There is no scientific way of determining the relative strength of the several arguments advanced to support the need for a rapid acceleration in the training of physicians and the countervailing propositions that have just been sketched. But the issue can be further explored. Here are some incisive comments made in passing at the recent conference that went unchallenged.

Many general surgeons are not busy, a fact which helps to explain why much unnecessary surgery continues to be performed. The situation with respect to hysterectomies is scandalous. We were told that many women undergo mastectomies when a less radical procedure would do. Likewise many thyroidectomies are performed where psychotherapy is indicated.

There is substantial overdoctoring for a host of diseases, including in particular infections of the upper respiratory tract, which constitute the single largest cause of morbidity. The indiscriminate prescribing of antibiotics was regarded as bad medicine and worse economics; nonetheless, this practice was recognized as being very widespread.

The major proponent of annual physical examinations was unable to convince his colleagues of its virtues. With the possible exception of the Papanicolaou test, screening devices, including even mass chest X-rays, were questioned. Without good follow-up procedures, screening appears to have limited value.

Although the potentialities of rehabilitation were not denied, we were reminded that only modest improvement could be expected from major efforts to help any large group of seriously stricken patients, such as victims of stroke.

The Conference agreed that excessive surgery, overdoctoring, and limitations of preventive medicine and rehabilitation are characteristic of the present state of medicine. And it was further agreed that the amount of medical services that a specific population group wants or needs depends, among other things, on its cultural background, education, and other traits. Hence, a preferred ratio of physicians to population in Boston or New York cannot be applied to the South—surely not to the rural South.

The observation was made that unsupervised residents and other less than fully qualified personnel are responsible for most of the physicians' services rendered in many large municipal and county hospitals. No one believed, however, that this defect could be eradicated simply by enlarging the output of medical schools. It was recognized that young physicians will be attracted to hospitals which have a strong teaching program and where a high quality of care is provided. To the extent that municipal and county hospitals are deficient on these scores, they will continue to experience great difficulty in attracting adequate staff.

While no one questioned the contention that the principal gains in health that the country has sustained since the beginning of this century have been due more to the rising standards of living and to advances in public health than to therapeutic medicine, the significance of this conclusion was not linked to discussions of future requirements for physicians. Similarly, when the conferees' attention was directed to the fact that in World War II the military withdrew about 40 percent of the physician manpower from the civilian community without causing much more than minor inconvenience to those who remained behind—in fact, the imperfect indices suggest that the public's health improved—they acknowledged the truth of the observation but failed to extend it.

Again, it was generally accepted that improved control over cigarette smoking, sexual promiscuity, and reckless driving offers potentially large gains in the public's health. But once again no connection was made between this fact and the limited role of physicians in achieving these objectives.

Similarly, while recognizing the desirability of rationalizing the delivery of medical services through the training and more effective use of allied health personnel the conferees did not apply this insight to modify their estimates of physician need. They knew, of course, that the marked gains in American medicine had been predicated during the past half century much more on improving the quality of the training of physicians than on a rapid increase in their numbers. And they also knew that the manpower requirements for the rapid expansion of the industry had been met essentially through the expansion of allied health manpower.

Much of the discussion reflecting the special interest and competence of the conferees was directed to ways in which the path through medical school and postgraduate medical education could be improved and shortened. Admission of selected students to medical school after two years of college, a three-year medical curriculum, elimination of internship, and reduction of various residencies from five to two years—all this and more was advanced and responded to favorably. It was clear that such reforms, if they were adopted, would add significantly to the potential supply of physicians. However, though each of these possibilities was noted and approved, there was no consensus that, individually or in total, they could significantly affect the estimated output of physicians. Possibly the conferees had no real confidence that one or more of these desirable changes were likely to occur in the near future on a scale that would have meaningful results.

So far the discussion has been limited to the arguments advanced by the proponents of a rapid step-up in the output of physicians and to the counter-arguments that denied that there was a crisis or that one was likely to develop even if special action to expand the supply were eschewed. However, a new dimension was introduced when a foundation president, not a physician, called attention to the anomalous situation in which fully qualified young men who desired to study medicine were unable to do so because of the limitation of training spaces. It was his contention that in a democracy, well-qualified persons should not be arbitrarily barred from pursuing a career of their choosing and he advanced this as a strong argument for expanding training facilities. The pressure to enter medical schools will inevitably mount in the decade ahead in the face of sharply rising undergraduate enrollments. To balance freedom of occupational choice, social investment in medical education, and the requirements for an efficient system of medical services will not come easily.

A rich society should be encouraged to give much weight to the ability of young people who are motivated and qualified to enter a profession of their own choosing. But this is a desideratum, not an overriding consideration. Aside from the substantial costs that are involved—most of which the society will presumably cover—the critical question that remains open is whether the additional physician manpower will be a boon. Most people, including the conferees, had no doubt on this score, but in fact the matter is not quite so uncomplicated.

For instance, physicians are in a position to determine their own demand. They usually have wide margins of discretion about whether to recommend that a patient return to the office for one or more follow-up visits. In short, physicians can, within broad limits, earn the income that they think they are entitled to earn.

Most economists believe that the public good would be served by a vast increase in the number of physicians which, through competition, would reduce average earnings and eliminate excessive gains from monopoly. Although no economist can look with equanimity on monopoly, in this instance the cure may be worse than the disease. If it is true that physicians can create their own demand, only a vast "oversupply" would bring average earnings down and the public would face the threat of being "overdoctored" as physicians sought to earn the income to which they believed themselves entitled. It may well be that the effective use of physician manpower depends in the first instance on a taut supply of physicians. Given the alternatives of high average earnings for a taut supply of physicians and a loose supply, lower fees, and overdoctoring, I opt unequivocally for the first.

This analysis has not led to definitive conclusions save one: No arbitrary figure is a proper guide for determining the desirable rate of expansion for the supply of physicians.

~ 8 ~

The Medical Specialist:
The Obstetrician

It is a characteristic of most professionals and even more so of most specialists to see the world from the special vantage point of their own field and to believe that their problems are unique; hence the solutions to them must be unique. However strong the forces pulling a society and an economy apart, it must be recognized that there are even stronger forces at work to relate the several parts to the whole. No institution plays a stronger role in the integrative function than the market place. As first described by Adam Smith, it functions to allocate men, money and other scarce resources in accordance with the priority demands of those who have money to spend.

On Money and Manpower

Few people realize that if a country decides to spend substantial sums on space research it will suddenly find itself short of space scientists; if it decides to spend substantial sums on economic research, it will suddenly find itself short of economists.

In recent years three tremendous sources of new funds have become available to medicine. One has been the federal government's large expenditures for medical research. Second, there has been the new money provided by Medicare and Medicaid. And third, as the American public becomes more affluent, the consumer has more money to spend. One might think that the consumer would prefer to buy other things than doctors' time, but apparently not.[1] Americans want to see more doctors, talk more with doctors, and generally have more to do with doctors. This being the case, it is not surprising that most people believe that there is a shortage of physicians. A safer formulation would be to talk of a taut supply.

An important characteristic of any professional service is the marked differences that exist, or that people believe exist, among the members authorized to provide the service. Only a very simple-minded person assumes that one physician is the equal of another. This being the case, increasing the total supply will never prevent those in a preferred market position from having preferred access to those with the most talent.

The U.S. Public Health Service has published data for many years on the distribution of physicians throughout the United States which prove that they tend to concentrate in the more affluent states. This was true in 1940. It is equally true in 1968.[2] If the number of physicians graduating in states with a preferred ratio of physicians to population increased very rapidly, some of the "excess" might spill over and relocate in areas where the ratio is less favorable. But it would require a tremendous increase in the supply to bring about any significant redistribution. And the leaders of the profession would not relocate.

The German Kasse system prior to World War II illustrated how medical services gravitate to those who can afford them. A physician working for the system of medical insurance might see 75 patients in the morning at a mark or so a visit but was likely to limit himself to 12 private patients in the afternoon. When there is a scarce good or service—and good doctors by definition are scarce, just like good actresses, good professors, good artists, and good mechanics—the people with more money will have preferred access to it.

The belief that we can bring about a situation in which everybody will have all the attention he desires and requires from qualified physicians is a delusion. Regardless of how many physicians a country has, such an outcome is unlikely. For example, Israel has more doctors per head of population than any other country in the world; there is more than one physician for every 500 persons. Nevertheless, rural coverage in Israel is inadequate; physicians do not want to live in the country. In Israel, the "country" is only an hour, at most two hours, from the city, but physicians balk at even this degree of separation from the urban environment.

This phenomenon of physicians concentrating in urban centers is worldwide. It is seen in such unlikely places as Ethiopia, where almost all of the three hundred resident physicians for a nation of about 25 million live in one of two cities, Addis Ababa or Asmara, and the socialist states of Eastern Europe, which have made strenuous efforts to broaden the access of the population, including the farm population, to health services. In Yugoslavia, recent medical school graduates accept employment as waiters or laborers in Belgrade in preference to an appointment as physician in a small town in the countryside. Much the same is true of Bulgaria, even though a young physician who accepts a rural position for a limited number of years will be able to accumulate considerable property and will have important professional preferment when he completes his period of duty.

The argument up to this point has stressed numerical ratios. If the focus were on specialists the result would be even more dramatic. The leaders of the medical profession throughout the world are city men who treat primarily the well-to-do.

On Medical Schools and Hospitals

Money and manpower are two of the three critical ingredients that determine the shape and functioning of a system of medical care. The third strategic element is the institutional framework within which the medical school and the hospital have come to play an ever more important role.

The medical school not only produces physicians, but its teaching hospital utilizes a disproportionate number of them. New medical schools are constantly being opened and our supply of physicians is being steadily expanded. But medical schools are peculiar. They use much medical manpower; they attract large numbers of residents. In obstetrics and gynecology, there are about three residents at hospitals affiliated with medical schools to one in a nonaffiliated hospital. In many teaching hospitals, interns and residents tumble over each other in an attempt to see a patient. However, they continue to flock to these hospitals in the knowledge that the training programs at university hospitals are superior.

We have a two-class system of hospitals in the United States—hospitals affiliated with a medical school and nonaffiliated hospitals. The anguish in this situation is reflected by the fact that Mount Sinai Hospital in New York City, a nationally renowned nonaffiliated hospital, saw no future for itself unless it could become affiliated with a strong medical school. Following several abortive efforts at university affiliation, it saw no alternative but to establish a new medical school under its own aegis.

Another aspect of the contemporary hospital's manpower problems relates to its heavy dependence on foreign-trained physicians for house staff. The university teaching hospital and the stronger community hospitals with good training programs or with sufficient funds to hire full-time house staff do not confront this issue. But a great many other large hospitals are able to cover their services only through employing large numbers of foreign-trained physicians. Since the focus of this chapter is on obstetrics and gynecology, it is worth noting that these services are on the average somewhat better off: only 1 in 5 is a foreign-trained physician in comparison to about 1 in 4 for most other specialties.[3]

While it is too early to assess the impact that Medicare and Medicaid will have on American medicine, no one questions that change is inevitable. Since poor people now have more money to spend on medicine, they are certain to do so. Moreover, since they now have a greater freedom of choice in seeking medical attention, they will doubtless avail themselves of it. It does not follow, however, that ignorant patients will necessarily choose wisely. A distinguished professor of medicine at Columbia University said many years ago that if he became ill in New York City, he would change his name and go on the ward of one of the large teaching hospitals. In the past, the indigent may not always have been handled with dignity but they often received good hospital care. The fact that patients will henceforth do the choosing is no guaranty that they will receive better treatment. Many of them will do worse when they trade the hard benches of the hospital clinic for the upholstered chairs in the outer office of the practitioners in the community, particularly in the ghetto.

The conviction of those who wrote the new legislation in Washington was that increasing the flow of money would inevitably improve the level of medical care. It may, but there is surely no certainty that it will. When physicians seek reimbursement from government for having treated 60 or 80 patients a day one cannot quiet the suspicion that most, if not all, of them have received perfunctory care.

American medicine is increasingly specialized medicine. We hear many voices in favor of resurrecting the general practitioner, of adding prestige and income to those who enter general practice, but the incontrovertible fact is that about 90 percent of all medical students look forward to becoming specialists. While some may change their minds and others will have their minds changed for them by circumstances, the overwhelming trend to specialization will not be reversed. This is a fact of advancing medical science with which we must live.

Another trend where the readings are confused relates to the evolving role of the hospital in the system of medical care. The hospital will continue to be the center where most of the dramatic advances in medicine will first be incorporated into the therapeutic system. But that is not enough. We have done little to correlate ambulatory with inpatient care. Medicare benefits for nursing-home care are conditioned on prior admission to a hospital. Logic and economy would dictate the opposite. Why force into a hospital patients who can be effectively treated as outpatients or in a nursing home?

We are a rich country and continue to become richer. And yet we are likely to face major financial difficulties in the health field within a few years because of our poor planning. Despite the large sums which government has added to the pool of medical purchasing power it is uncertain how many patients are really better off. Admittedly Medicare is a boon to old people. Within the past two years, leading hospitals in New York City have increased their charges from about $50 per day for a room to $100. After the passage of Medicaid, many hospitals succeeded in raising their per diem reimbursement from government from about $50 to about $90. Yet, these hospitals provide about the same service this year that they gave last year. But the public is paying 80 percent more. The preferred explanation of hospital administrators for these increases are salary adjustments for the poorly paid staff. There is merit to this but it falls short of a complete explanation.

Another intriguing problem that bears directly both on the quality of medical care available to the people who live in New York City, as well as on the effectiveness with which medical manpower is utilized, is grounded in the dual hospital system—voluntary and municipal—that is characteristic of the nation's largest metropolis. As several experts and commissions, particularly in Western Pennsylvania and Rochester, New York, have indicated, inadequate community control over the erection and expansion of hospital beds can contribute significantly to raising hospital bills. This difficulty is compounded in New York City, which supports two parallel systems coordinated only at the fringes. Moreover, coordination takes place only when it leads to a clear advantage to the voluntary group. Although the issue has been in the public domain at least since the late 1940s, nobody has yet found the political nostrum that would speed the integration of the two and insure that the total expenditures for hospital care resulted in a reasonable level of care for all patients, affluent and poor alike. It may be too early to draw firm conclusions from our experience with Medicare and Medicaid, but the substantial infusion of new governmental dollars will probably do little, if anything, to improve matters. Before the recent (1968) reductions in Medicaid it looked as if there might be a substantial shift in the work load from municipal to voluntary hospitals as the poor could cover their costs of hospital care. But such drift as took place ceased and was probably reversed when the funds for Medicaid were cut back. And even if the trend away from the municipal system had continued, it is by no means clear that the poor would have benefited.

The situation in many hospital clinics remains disturbing. They do not operate efficiently and yet some are now seeking reimbursement from government of up to $25.00 a visit! Specialists on Park Avenue are willing to see patients for a comparable fee. We are watching raids on the public purse about which the public is not yet fully aware, but the truth cannot long remain hidden.

A neglected aspect of medical care relates to minority groups. The Negro poor probably receive less adequate care than the Puerto Rican poor because of the greater insecurities and hostilities that characterize the Negro community. There is scattered evidence to support the statement that Puerto Ricans make somewhat better use of available medical facilities. Some Negroes have probably tended to avoid white physicians and white hospitals in the present stage of race relationships. But with relatively few well-qualified Negro physicians in active practice and with their numbers not likely to increase rapidly, many Negroes fail to receive the medical help they require. One optimistic note is that the allied health professions are proving attractive, particularly to Negro women.

It looked for a time as if the innovative, federally financed community health centers which placed substantial responsibility on local leadership for planning the services to be provided and for hiring and supervising the staff might be a mass solution, although high costs and man-power problems posed immediate obstacles. But the closing of the federal spigot means that the number of such centers will be quite limited. They will surely not be the answer to the Negroes' overall need for better medical services.

What we find, therefore, is much new money flowing into the financing of medical services resulting in some significant gains for older people and better compensation for lowly paid hospital workers. But when we take a closer look at the operation of hospitals and clinics, particularly their provision of services for the poor, there is little basis for optimism. Some things have changed, but much has not. And all of the changes have not been for the good.

On Obstetrics and Obstetricians

The practice of obstetrics is particularly vulnerable to the changing contours of urban life with its radical shifts of population. Nowhere is this more true than in New York City, particularly in Brooklyn. During the decade of the 1950s, about 1.25 million whites left the city. The homes and apartments that they vacated were filled in con-siderable measure with new immigrants from the South and Puerto Rico, most of whom could not afford a private physician or specialist. Hence obstetricians were faced with the loss of paying patients. But that is not the end of the difficulty. The principal teaching hospitals which had the responsibility for providing care for the poor were faced with unbalanced staff. A large institution such as Brooklyn's Kings County Hospital found that most of its residents fled the city once they had completed their training. These and other manpower distortions may help to explain some shocking epidemiological facts.

According to the reports of the Department of Health, about a quarter of all women delivered in New York City have no prenatal care or are seen by a doctor only just prior to delivery. In the Bedford-Stuyvesant area, the figure is 40 percent; 2 out of every 5 women do not see a physician until they are close to the end of their pregnancy. In Bay Ridge, by contrast, the percentage is about 8. Money is part of the explanation, but education, cultural attitudes, and location play a role, as does the availability of physician manpower.

Nobody will argue that it is bad for a woman to see a physician regularly during her pregnancy, although uncertainty remains about the precise relationship between prenatal care and maternal and infant health. Presumptively prenatal care is better than non-care. But one thing we do know: neonatal death rates for different groups vary greatly; those for Bedford-Stuyvesant are twice as high as for other parts of the borough.

Pregnancy is a condition, not a disease, and except where there are complications, the margins of difference due to intervention are likely to be small. In the absence of abnormality we can expect a natural process to reach termination without difficulty. This fact helps to explain why Kings County Hospital can safely release its obstetrical patients after 36 hours while many other hospitals keep them six days or longer, and why in Holland, for example, most deliveries take place not in the hospital, but at home. Most women deliver normally. Some develop complications and these are the ones who require special attention and care. Neither pregnancy nor birth is pathological.

The Department of Health reports that in 1965, there were only 16 therapeutic abortions for every 10,000 births in New York City. That is a shocking statistic since many psychotic and mentally defective women become pregnant. If we were primarily concerned with the health of the community, a significant part of the efforts of obstetricians and gynecologists would be devoted to educating the public and educating the legislature about the importance not only of reducing the neonatal death rate but also of insuring that certain pregnancies do not eventuate in a live birth.

A member of a recent presidential task force, a conservative businessman, argued that it is the natural and inalienable right of every woman to decide whether she wants to have a baby or not. Another distinguished member of the group, a professor of law, was asked what he thought the chances were that the Supreme Court would uphold this view. To the amazement of most of the members of the task force, the law professor indicated that in his view a strong case could be made to support the contention that every woman has the right to determine whether or not to have a child and that at some time in the future the Supreme Court would so decide. Because of the deep moral and religious issues involved, however, he added that the Court would certainly avoid hearing such a case for some years.

While reliable figures are not available it is clear that the general practitioner's role in obstetrical care has been diminishing and will continue to do so. But it is also clear that many women, particularly those from low-income and minority groups, receive very little medical attention prior to and after delivery. Hence there are leaders in the profession who have argued in favor of developing a professional sub-specialty of nurse-midwives, convinced that they can provide a high level of obstetrical care for all except a small minority of women who have complications. This is the general structure of obstetrical care in most European countries where medical science is almost as sophisticated, and health standards at least as high as in the United States.[4]

Reasonable as the proposal sounds, it is doubtful that it will gain general acceptance. With the growth in power and influence of the medical profession and the development of specialization in obstetrics, midwifery, which was widely practiced early in this century, fell into disrepute and persisted only among first generation immigrant groups, southern Negroes, and some isolated rural communities. Only 1.3 percent of all live births in 1966 were reported as attended by midwives.[5] Midwives have been forced out of the pattern of medicine in the United States, and the outlook for their return as independent practitioners is not auspicious. However, experiments in the utilization of nurse-midwives within the hospital team are progressing, and these nurse specialists may make a substantial contribution to more effective service within the framework of hospital-based and group-practice obstetrics.

A particularly interesting aspect of obstetrics to the student of manpower is that few practitioners grow old at their work. At some point obstetrical practice becomes too wearing and the physician is forced to shift, usually to gynecology. But this leads to the difficult question of whether there is enough gynecological work for the specialists as well as the shifters.

A knowledgeable leader of medicine in the Middle West recently reported that tired obstetricians were a major source of supply for the large number of medical planners required under the several new pieces of federal legislation. However ill-equipped they may be for this new role, it may be preferable to absorb them here than to force them to earn their livelihoods by practicing surgery.

We now face in the arena of medical care what we faced earlier in medical research. Large sums of new money have been introduced into a system which is characterized by relatively high inelasticity of its key resource—the competent physician. There are no easy answers to this dilemma, once it has been created. Many argue that the dilemma exists only in the eye of the critic. What possible way was there to increase the quantity and quality of medical research but to make large sums available and assume that with time the research capabilities of the country would expand to cope with the new opportunities? Similarly, many argue that there is no better way of assuring that the poor and the aged achieve access to better medical care than to provide them with the resources to pay for it. There is much to be said for this simplistic approach to the restructuring of our medical system.

But it may be a little too simple. In obstetrics, for example, whether midwives have a future in American medicine depends on much more than the availability of funds; the inevitability of obstetricians having to reduce or give up their practices as they get older is likewise not a question of money; whether they should perform more therapeutic abortions; and whether at the time of delivery they should prevent many women from having additional children, all have little to do with money per se.

Clearly money plays a critical role in attracting medical resources and in determining their allocation and use. But simply adding to the amount of purchasing power of the American people for health care is no guarantee that it will be adequate either in amount or quality and even less that it will be distributed according to need.

～9～

New Missions
for Public Health

One way to begin an evaluation of the manpower problems of public health is to set it within a larger framework of the aims and goals of the field.

Nutrition has long been an area of major concern to public health. However, when children were organized into work groups in Watts and given simple assignments, several fainted from hunger. Much has been written about the inability of the ghetto child to learn in school. But not many public health officials appreciate the remark of Ellen Winston, U.S. Commissioner of Welfare, at the White House Conference on Education in 1965, that hungry children cannot learn. Nor can sleepy children.

In Watts, girls of 16 or 17 are pregnant and have youngsters in their arms or toddling beside them. Family planning, along with nutrition, is within the province of public health.

We all know that public health should play a role in community psychiatry and community mental health. But public health officials have not paid attention to the fact that Negro boys in the poorest sections of the ghetto—two-thirds of whom come from families in which there is no father—are taught in school by women. This must be reflected in psychic development and mental health.

The only community-wide facility in Watts prior to the 1965 riots was a public health clinic. But the staff did not disseminate what they had learned to those in a position of power who might have been able to help.

These introductory comments about Watts are a reminder of the gap between goals and accomplishments in public health that are all too visible within one ghetto of a rich and populous state. As the discussion shifts to manpower, it would be well to relate resources to returns. We can begin with a consideration of some specific manpower approaches formulated by a distinguished leader of the profession:

Massive development of subprofessional
aides and assistants

This is a sensible way for a field that is short of trained professionals to move but, as nursing has shown, it is not a panacea. Even if large numbers of subprofessionals can be recruited and trained in public health, they will leave the field unless they have reasonable career opportunities. One of the handicaps of most health fields, including public health, is the absence of career opportunities for those with modest education and training.

There is an additional reason to be wary. The effective use of subprofessional personnel implies that direction and supervision by professionals will be adequate. In this connection, how much of the education and training of professionals in public health is focused on teaching them to supervise subprofessionals?

*Development of new technologies with
consequent new positions and titles*

The answer does not lie in opening up a large number of new positions with new titles related to new techniques and new functions that grow out of the new technologies. Public health faces the more serious challenge of rethinking its goals, reassessing its resources, and realigning its methods in a broad *systems* approach.

There are problems, however, on this front. It has long been the aspiration and conviction of the public health physician that he should be the leader of the health team. In some regards this is sound. But as the field of public health has developed, there are many areas where others who are not physicians are likely to be more competent. A basic issue is to assure that the best qualified professional is at the helm.

*More rapid expansion of recruitment and of
training resources*

Probably public health is right in wanting both more and better recruitment and training, but recruitment means the same to the manpower planner as patriotism does to the scoundrel. If one cannot solve his problems with the manpower at hand, what is more logical than to ask for additional manpower?

Training not geared to promotion and career advancement is likely to contribute not to more effective utilization but to frustration and resignations. Why should a man undertake training unless he can profit from it?

These are tentative approaches now in vogue which attempt to deal more effectively with the manpower challenges facing public health. It is questionable, however, that we can deal intelligently with the question of manpower without raising, antecedently, the question of goals.

Here are eight critical points:

1. Almost every field dependent on trained manpower complains about manpower shortages. In instances where government funds have been vastly increased, the shortages are more acute because they have been engendered by appropriating money more quickly than people can be trained. From this point of view the manpower "crisis" in public health is far from unique.

Some will agree that it was fortunate that Congress was less enthusiastic about public health than about therapeutic medicine; otherwise public health would have received even more funds and today would have even more severe manpower problems.

2. Every field, including public health, will fail to solve its manpower needs if it insists upon perpetuating long-established patterns of staffing. The key to economic progress is through increases in productivity. In areas where capital cannot readily be substituted for manpower, as in the health services, a critical way of making productivity gains is through shifting resources from lower to higher priority goals.

We cannot simply keep adding new objectives to existing ones without getting rid of others, especially since it is often no longer necessary to perpetuate certain types of services.

For instance, some years ago public health was concerned with a public that had average of less than eight grades of education. Today, young people are entering adulthood with an average of one year of post-high-school education. Such a change must make it possible for public health to reduce or eliminate certain programs to which it previously had devoted resources, such as teaching a college graduate how to bathe her newborn.

3. Every field, including public health, finds the shifting of goals and redirection of resources difficult to achieve because of organizational inflexibility, conservative professional attitudes, and weakness in leadership. Yet unless changes are made, the manpower crisis can never be relieved.

Every professional organization operates for the benefit of its members, which means that the leadership is restricted in what it can do. An extreme formulation would be that the struggle is frequently between the aims and goals of the membership of a professional organization and the needs and desires of the public. Frequently the public has little chance of getting its needs met because of the strength of the professional organization.

4. The fact that public health is such a fragmented field, with semiautonomous units in control of limited resources focused on specific goals, makes the problem of reform more difficult, yet more essential. The more dynamic the

field, the more difficult it is to reform. While retraining offers one way of bringing older personnel and new functions into closer alignment, retraining is not the key. It is not possible, generally, to take a physician with a quarter of a century's experience in contagious diseases and turn him into an expert in nuclear medicine.

5. Failure to redefine goals and to shift the resources required to meet them also implies an unsatisfactory articulation with the education and training of manpower. It seems questionable that because physicians were asked to head many fields of public health when communicable diseases had a priority role, this pattern should persist when such problems as medical economics, hospital administration, and water and air pollution are high on the list. A rethinking of staffing requirements, pursuant to a shifting of goals, is urgently required. And this implies corresponding adjustments in the educational structure.

Those who teach know about the inevitability of a lag between optimal practice and standard instruction. Tension between the two is always present. If outmoded staffing and antiquated procedures remain in effect in the field, the spread between practice and the schools can increase to a point where the lag in the educational structure may widen from one generation to two.

6. In the past, public health has fought a losing battle with therapeutic medicine for the delivery of medical services. Perhaps it would be the better part of wisdom for public health to recognize that it is unlikely to win, even with Titles XVIII and XIX of the Medicare Act. If it stops advancing claims to direct medical service programs

and concentrates its efforts on planning and evaluation, public health might have a better chance for significant accomplishment. A field that attempts too much will fail to achieve what it might accomplish if it harnessed its resources more effectively.

It is by no means clear that public health should enlarge or even perpetuate independent operation of service programs. After all, it has long had responsibility for control of tuberculosis, venereal disease, infant mortality, accidents, and for health education, particularly in the fields of nutrition and smoking. A reading of the performance record does not make clear that this is an optimal framework for the execution even of such traditional public health service responsibilities.

7. In the presence of continuing shortages of trained manpower, public health might best realize certain high-priority goals by developing effective coordinating devices with other professions in a position to help—scientists and engineers interested in problems of pollution and accident control, and such diverse groups as educators, welfare officials, employment officials, and the clergy, each of whom might be able to help in realizing one or another major health objective—from family planning to the control of diet and smoking.

The importance of coordination, horizontally and vertically, is seen in Watts. It makes little sense if the public health worker in such an area is not closely associated with other professionals engaged in seeking to provide services to children and adults. Individually, each is likely to have little influence or impact. Collectively, there is at least a chance that they might be able to affect the shape of things.

8. In a society increasingly aware of community needs and committed to social welfare, public health should be an exciting field full of challenges. As such, it should be able to attract a reasonable proportion of able people. But it will be able to do so only if it succeeds in reorganizing itself to increase the efficiency with which it does its work.

If the principal way into a satisfactory career in public health continues to be through the medical school, the numbers who will find their way into public health will remain relatively small. While physicians should continue to be in control of certain facets of the work, it does not follow that they must be in control of all of it.

Public health urgently needs a rethinking of its functions and of the appropriate types and levels of training for those who will carry the primary responsibilities. It is also important to build multiple bridges so that individuals with less training who are interested and motivated can enhance their skills and move up to higher level work.

The foregoing dicta can be reformulated thus. In a dynamic society time produces changes, and the institutions that were brought into being at an earlier period to cope with particular problems will find that some, often many, of their tasks have in fact been eroded by alterations in the environment and in the priority needs of the population. Concurrently, time brings to the fore new challenges with which established institutions will be unable to cope unless they secure additional resources of men and money. But it is clearly impossible to add indefinitely to the resources of established institutions so as to enable them to cope more effectively with the new. Other adjustments can and must be made:

Certain functions can be eliminated.

Certain functions can be merged.

Certain functions can be reassigned to personnel with lesser competence.

Certain functions can be performed with less manpower and more capital.

Certain functions can be transferred from the provider to the consumer of the service.

Certain functions can be carried out by persons with less training.

Unless the leadership of a profession is able to accomplish the foregoing, the institutions which they head will soon become dysfunctional: they will be engaged in tasks of lesser importance carried over from the past; and they will be unable to secure the resources of manpower and money to respond effectively to new high-priority demands.

No matter how many reforms are introduced, however, it is likely that a manpower stringency will continue. Most people look on such a situation as a bane. It can also be a boon. The one sure way to waste skills, to discourage trained people, to disenchant staff, is to have enough people for all the work that needs doing. Then nobody will be able to stretch—for if he does, he will impinge on somebody else's prerogatives and functions. If there is a shortage of people, then, and only then, will the latent and developed potentials of people be fully utilized.

Public health does not face a crisis in manpower. It faces a crisis in being.

๏ 10 ๏

The Woman Physician

In the census of physicians, women account for about 8 percent of the total; extended to the total field of health manpower, the woman physician is reduced to a minute statistic, less than a tenth of a tenth.[1] Given the revolution in female labor power and in the health services industry, an analysis of this phenomenon of small numbers might best be approached through several interrelated areas: important trends in the professions; facts about women who work; and the structural characteristics of the medical field and its manpower dimensions. Against the background of these more general considerations, the focus will narrow to women in medicine, with the major concern of relating analysis to policy.

The most significant fact that emerges from any overview of the professions is that in the United States today they constitute the fastest growing segment of the total labor force. Employment in professional occupations has increased faster than in any other category; in the last fifteen years, the number of people in the professions has more than doubled. Yet the curious thing is that over the last quarter century, the proportion of women in the professions has not changed. It remains at a stable 13 percent.

A second significant fact is that the professions have become more intensely professional. In the pre-World War II days a professional degree could be obtained in fewer years and marked the end of the education and training process for the professional. Today it is only the beginning. In many fields, particularly in research, post-doctoral work is virtually mandatory. There is progressively more specialization within each profession. And that has had an important built-in time effect: the number of years preempted for education relative to the number of income-producing years is approaching 1 to 2.

In addition, the monetary costs of obtaining a degree keep rising. Universities have found it necessary to keep increasing their tuition charges. While state and federal scholarship and fellowship aid has moderated this burden it is still onerous for many students. For various and complex reasons, one of which has been the unyielding opposition of the American Medical Association, broad federal financial assistance to medical students has not been made possible. The net result has been that a physician's education is increasingly costly.

While young physicians can earn sizable incomes shortly after obtaining their licenses, most will not because they are likely to spend, in addition to two years in military service, three to five years in qualifying as specialists.

Another point is the critical importance of continuing education. Today no physician can remain professionally alive unless he has the opportunity of continuing to study while he is working. Yet the structure of the profession deters him. One of the weaknesses of our medical system is that it is structured upon a broad base of private practitioners who have to stop earning if they wish to keep studying. And the educational structure is only just beginning to design programs to accommodate the practitioner.

The overall costs in time and money of a professional education are not all that have been changing; the students, their needs, and their demands are also changing. Today's university student has commitments beyond the lecture room and the lab: he is characteristically married and often a parent besides. This is a new phenomenon. Professional education, marriage, a family—formerly these were sequential; today education and marriage coincide.

The general pattern of early marriage in this country has particular significance for women students. With so many of their friends marrying early, many girls who are still in college or graduate school do not want to delay making a marital choice. The competition extends even to starting a family early.

Further importance attaches to the marked increase of opportunities in the realm of the professions and related academic areas. Until recently, there were four classic professions: medicine, law, the army, and the clergy. Now there is a proliferation of professional fields, with particular elaboration in the sciences—all competing vigorously for the gifted college student. Medicine faces many new and attractive competitors.

Against this brief review of the professions, let us consider certain characteristics of women who work, since this is another parameter of the problem. It is true today—and it is likely to be true tomorrow—that more and more

women work, and they will work for more years of their
lives. Admittedly, farm women have always worked and
they have worked hard. But in the transition from a farm
to an industrial society most married women did not work
out of the home. The change came during World War II.
Today women are likely to be outside the labor force only
during the years when they are raising their children, or
when they are old or sick. The work pattern of women is
likely to resemble more and more that of men. This is a
clear break with the recent past.

A few figures can help to make this point. Fifty percent
of all women aged 45 to 55 are now employed. Thus it is
the older women, even more than the younger ones, who
are most likely to be working. In years past, the Army, for
one, had a rule that women past the age of 40 were not to
be sent overseas; the years after 40 were assumed to be
high-risk years for women, fraught with nervousness and
instability. Today there is great regard for the middle-aged
female worker.

Another interesting and telling characteristic of the
working woman is the extent of her education. In general,
the more education a woman has, the more likely she is to
work. The data are unequivocal. Two-thirds of all women
who have had at least one year of graduate study are working. That is, at any time, two-thirds of all women who
have completed five years of higher education are in the
labor force. This proportion diminishes for those with less
education. With only a bachelor's degree, for instance, the
percentage employed drops to 45 percent. Clearly, the more

investment a woman makes in study, the more likely she is
to put that investment to work.[2]

However, a high proportion of women work part time
throughout the year, or full time for part of the year. Only
a minority of working women, 2 out of 5, work full time,
full year.[3] Now that has serious implications, particularly
for women who contemplate a professional career.

One of the more interesting findings is that over the last
decade or so the pace of women's reentry into the labor
force has quickened; women do not have to wait until they
are 45 to go back to work. The younger age groups are returning to the work force in larger numbers, and the more
education they have, the less time they are content to remain out of the labor force. The data suggest that more
and more women wish to continue to work even while they
have young children at home, and this tendency is re-
enforced with increased educational achievement.

Although women receive over 40 percent of all baccalaureate degrees conferred in the United States, and the
percentage is rising, they receive only 32 percent of all
master's degrees, a proportion that has remained constant
for many years. At the doctoral level, however, there has
been a radical drop. From 15 percent in 1920, the proportion of women doctorate recipients decreased to 9 percent
in 1950, and only gradually was restored to 11 percent by
1960, where it has stabilized. Since World War II, efforts
at motivating a higher proportion of women to continue
to the doctorate apparently have had little effect. Their
distribution varies greatly by academic field, from a mini-

mum in the sciences to a creditable 20 percent or more in education, the arts, and the humanities.[4]

Other factors than numbers have also changed. Before World War II, a high proportion of the women who earned a doctorate were single-minded careerists. They were determined to find their place in the scheme of things as professionals and academicians, and they were not at all concerned with the complicating problems of husband, family, and other responsibilities. Thirty years ago, a distinguished woman scientist, a Radcliffe graduate, even though she married late, was regarded as a traitor to her class when she did. Attitudes and life styles are different today.

The majority of women physicians currently marry colleagues or men in allied fields. This has economic implications. The high professional income of her husband correlates negatively with a woman's likelihood to work, certainly to work at maximal capacity.

Here are a few salient facts about the medical profession. The basic image of the medical practitioner in our American culture is masculine. It is difficult work; it is a harsh, demanding life; it requires physical strength, emotional imperturbability, and hard-nosed logic—and these characteristics we associate with men.

Related are the specific sexual attitudes of the American public which has reservations about the propriety of physical examination and treatment of adult males by female physicians. There is little objection to receiving ophthalmologic care from women, and female pediatricians and psychiatrists may even have special appeal in our current

climate of gentleness. Many women patients prefer obstetrical and gynecologic care by a woman physician. This
undoubtedly accounts for the heavy concentration of
women in these specialties. However, any program to encourage the greater representation of women in other
arenas of medical practice must take account of overt and
covert attitudes of patients, medical educators, and even
prospective students. These are not readily dissipated.[5]

Normally one enters medical school after having majored in science in college. With regard to teachers of science, one of two statements probably is valid: Some are
disappointed because they were unable to go into medicine
and they may work out some of their disappointments on
their students. Others are proselytizing on behalf of their
own field of specialization. It is not difficult to understand
that an able professor of biology might challenge a bright
woman student: "Why do you want to go into medicine?
It is dull, dreary, and you will be looking down people's
throats or pulling out splinters. Here you have the whole
of science as your future domain."

Another relevant point about contemporary medicine in
the United States is its predominantly private entrepreneurial structure. The aggressiveness required for successful solo practice, the competitiveness, the limited possibilities for allocating or deputizing basic responsibility—all are
potential sources of conflict for a life style that combines
family and profession. In the selection of a career these
conditions are likely to deter a good number of even
strongly motivated women students.

As the difficult terms of our system of private practice

discourage women from entering medicine, the potentially high earnings of the field reinforce masculine prejudices against facilitating their entry into the profession. Income potential is an important factor that operates to maintain the highly preferred position of medicine in the spectrum of career options for men, and this will not easily be ceded to women. The converse is seen in the related field of nursing: viewed traditionally as a female profession, wages persisted at a low level for a long period, and nursing has never attracted men.

The continuing elongation of medical training, which is the educational concomitant of the inexorable advance of specialization, has especially serious implications for prospective women physicians. Family and career compete for the same prime years, and by and large medicine has failed to accommodate to the dual commitment of women. Education, graduate and undergraduate, and, to a lesser extent, practice are rigidly structured for full-time activity. This is consistent with the work patterns of the adult male in our society, but it is not congenial to female participation. There is no flexibility at the undergraduate level and only the bare beginnings at the graduate level. True, internships and residencies are somewhat less full time than before: house staff is no longer required to sleep in, and 8 hours has replaced 24 hours as the standard on-duty shift. Nevertheless, house staff positions remain basically full time, justified by hospital needs more than educational desiderata, and they are harsh for women.

Finally, the student capacity of our medical schools, which is increasing at only a moderate rate, places an upper bound on the potential of any effort to encourage a greater acceptance of women, despite the universally assumed shortage of physicians. Even with additional places in each succeeding first-year class, the ratio of applicants to places *nationwide* is now at more than 2:1, and by all accounts student applicants are for the most part fully qualified.[6] We are likely to see an increasing number of applicants for demographic reasons: the pool of 22-year-olds, from whom the freshman class of professional schools is drawn, reflects the enlarged birth rates after 1946. The inroads into the graduate student pool caused by demands of the draft are also likely to impel many bright college men toward a medical career. Given both enhanced admissions pressures and enhanced demand pressures for practicing physicians, how likely are medical schools to liberalize admissions and academic policies in order to attract larger numbers of women who are already considered attrition risks both at school and in the profession?

The regional pattern underlying the expansion of medical schools is, on the whole, favorable to women applicants. We find that the medical schools in the Northeast—New England through Pennsylvania—produce 40 percent of all the women physicians in the country, while they graduate only 30 percent of all physicians. In other words, the more emancipated East contributes disproportionately to the supply of women physicians. The Midwest, which produces just about the same proportion of all physicians as the East, produces only 20 percent of women physicians. The rest of the country is pretty much in balance.

Against this background it is worth noting where the

new medical schools are being established. They are at Arizona, Brown, Davis, La Jolla, Connecticut, Hawaii, Louisiana State, Michigan State, Mount Sinai (New York), Stony Brook, Penn State, Rutgers, Texas South, and Toledo State. Of these, only two are Midwestern schools—Michigan State and Toledo State. This means that the region of the country which has failed to pull its weight in the training of women physicians is accounting for only a small part of the expanded capacity.

The East has produced more than its proportional share and will continue to do so. This augurs well for an increasing proportion of women in medicine.

The foregoing analysis leads directly into policy suggestions for the expanded participation and more effective utilization of women in the medical field, where scientific orientation is displacing clinical orientation, but which is embarrassed by its inability to satisfy mounting clinical demands.

The patterns of practice of women physicians reveal significant differences from those of men, and these may suggest potential avenues of adjustment. Only half of the women actively engaged in medicine are in private practice, compared with more than 75 percent of the men. Traditionally, it has been maintained, chiefly in justification of resistance to the admission of more women into medicine, that, given a professional education equal to that of men, they are less productive. While their efficiency and quality have never been assailed, it is true that women physicians work significantly less than their male colleagues. Even if we disregard the larger proportion of inactive women physicians, the active male doctor works at his career an average of one-third longer than the female. In a period of stringent supply, it is difficult to overlook these factors in the competition for medical school admission.

A case could be made for relieving some of the shortages in specialized fields by adjusting training programs, which are essentially full time, to the needs of women for less than full-time work, particularly in the early graduate years. Several areas, conspicuously psychiatry, pediatrics, and public health, have devised residencies that women can more readily undertake. Others, including general surgery, obstetrics and gynecology, ENT and ophthalmology, have not provided part-time programs and clearly do not wish to encourage any but the most unencumbered and dedicated women to enter.

Financing a medical education may also constitute a special deterrent to women. There now are loan programs, but not many young women contemplate entering a marriage with debts, a negative dowry so to speak, or with the need to postpone having a family. This is much more burdensome to women students than to men.

A final point concerns the limited mobility of physicians. Awareness of the chronic and increasing dearth of physician services for certain groups in our population—our rural population and the minorities in our urban ghettos—frequently elicits the hopeful statement that increasing the supply of women may relieve the shortage. However, the truth is that women will not be distributed any more equitably than the men they marry. Recent figures indicate that

Russia, where medicine has been predominantly a female profession, is reducing the proportion of women medical students. This may well be an attempt to correct physician maldistribution. There, as here, professional women marry professional men, frequently specialists, who tend to be concentrated in the cities.

Withal, the surprising fact is that there has been a significant gain in the involvement of women in American medical schools. During the last decade or so, the proportion of women in medicine has moved from 5 to over 8 percent and while we are dealing with small numbers, that is actually a 60 percent increase in a relatively short period of time. That is a clear trend.

How can it be encouraged? Any policies which would facilitate entrance into medicine, such as revisions in education and training structure, would be favorable for women students. We do not know whether basic changes will occur, or how soon, but they would be desirable. Some differentiation of medical training which would offer the possibility of qualifying for practice short of the present excessive period of time would be effective. Easier financing of a professional education would be an inducement. Today only the relatively wealthy can invest in a lengthy education; to the middle class and lower middle class the financial problem is very real; and to the lower class it presents an almost insuperable obstacle. The expansion of medical school facilities will mean a larger proportion of training opportunities for women only to the extent that it is accompanied by greater adaptability of program and curriculum. More effective utilization of women in actual medical practice is likely to come about with organizational changes in the system of health care. Group practice, salaried positions, and less than full-time jobs employ disproportionate numbers of women today, and their expansion will provide further attractive opportunities.

These will, however, constitute only minor adjustments. Far more basic sociological changes will be required before women in any large numbers exercise their theoretical option to enter medicine as freely as they enter other professions, such as teaching and intellectual fields, such as the humanities and arts. Career predilections are culturally determined and our culture conceives of medicine in terms of the male doctor. Career options close out early, certainly not much later than secondary school. We must consciously work to keep them open as long as possible, and we must direct our efforts at influencing them at the point when they are still real. Educational counseling and particularly curriculum choices are critical determinants, and it is upon these potentially powerful instruments that we might well focus in an attempt to effect real change.

PART THREE
Allied Health
Manpower

❧ II ❧

The Expanding Supply

The drama of medicine is centered around the physician who, from the depth of his expertise, can diagnose the cause of the patient's illness and act to relieve his symptoms by removing the causes of his disability. This is how the layman sees the situation and this is how the physician has helped him to understand contemporary medicine.

But the facts are somewhat different. One of the important contributions that Harry Greenfield and Carol Brown have made in their new book, *Allied Health Manpower: Trends and Prospects,* is to provide a comprehensive view of the manpower dimensions of contemporary American medicine and, without denigrating the strategic role of the physician, to shed new light on the approximately 2.5 million persons who, together with the slightly more than 300,000 physicians, are engaged in the provision of health services.[1] The authors are not primarily concerned with the relatively small numbers of independent practitioners such as dentists and other core professionals, nor even with the approximately 300,000 allied health professionals who have been trained between the baccalaureate and the doctoral levels and who fill such critical positions as bacteriologist, mycologist, biostatistician, virologist, hospital administrator, or clinical psychologist. Rather, their focus is on the approximately 1.7 million health workers who have been categorized as "allied health manpower," a reflection of the fact that they have one characteristic in common: all of them have had less than a full college education. While the majority are high-school graduates with some college training, a sizable number, probably over half a million, have not finished high school.

The single largest subgroup within allied health manpower are registered nurses who have graduated from a diploma school or from a junior college. They account for over half a million. But since nursing has been repeatedly singled out for study in depth, and since still another large-scale study is currently under way, the authors have devoted their attention primarily to the 1.2 million other health workers who fall within the rubric of allied health manpower. This large grouping contains five categories of technicians: x-ray, medical records, occupational therapy, medical, and dental; and three large categories of assistants: licensed practical nurses, nurse's aides, and psychiatric aides.

It may be helpful to set out briefly the major characteristics of these allied health workers and the major trends that can be identified with respect to their recruitment and utilization. This will provide a solid base from which to explore alternative public policies for more effectively utilizing this large and important group to provide essential health services for the American people.

As to their characteristics: reference has already been made to their level of education, which ranges from less than elementary school completion to just short of college graduation. The median level is one year of college. The overwhelming majority, about 4 out of 5, are women, who tend to be composed of two subgroups: those in their late teens, and those in their late thirties or above. The fact that about 40 percent of all women workers in the field are under 35 years of age suggests that many health workers tend to drop out of the labor force after a few years and start to raise families. Many come back, part time or full time, but usually not until their youngest child is in school.

Reliance on large numbers of modestly educated young female workers who remain at work for a limited number of years helps to explain the proliferation of training programs, particularly those which present short courses. Since health training below the professional level is only slowly being integrated into the formal educational system—that is, in vocational and comprehensive high schools and in junior and senior colleges—hospitals and other large medical institutions have had to train their own recruits. Much of the training has been short and of indifferent quality— just enough to enable the newcomer to carry out certain limited functions under strict supervision.

The heavy reliance of the health services industry on female labor also helps to explain the relatively low wage rates that have prevailed and which continue to prevail in most regions of the country. Men stay away from jobs which offer little prospect of income sufficient to support a family at a modest level even after many years of work. And the relatively small number of men in the allied health occupations operates to depress the wage scales.

These tendencies have been compounded by federal and state legislation which have excluded hospital employees from the provisions of fair labor standards acts and which further interdicted the unionization of hospital workers. While recent changes have occurred on both fronts, wages and working conditions in the health services industry continue to lag behind the more advanced sectors of the economy.

Despite these shortcomings and lags, the industry was able to expand its work force rapidly during the recent past. Between 1950 and 1965, employees on nonagricultural payrolls increased by one-third—from 45 to 60 million. During the same period, total medical manpower increased from 1.5 to 2.8 million, or by 87 percent, that is, two and a half times the rate for the economy as a whole.

Several factors contributed to this growth. First, the last two decades have witnessed rapid increases in the overall proportion of women who are actively engaged in remunerative employment, and the health services industry has been traditionally hospitable to women workers. Moreover, hospitals were able to absorb large numbers of unskilled workers, and many of the women who sought employment were unskilled. Next, hospitals located in the large urban centers found that the only prospect of their securing the large numbers of workers they required to meet their replacement and expansion needs was through abandoning their racially discriminatory practices. The health services industry began to attract ever larger numbers of minority group members. This tendency was reinforced by the thrust of recent federal manpower programs which placed heavy emphasis on health training for minority group members.

There is only one way to read the record. Despite the embryonic state of health planning, despite the inherent difficulties of managing a hospital because of the insistence of physicians to have their own way, despite the hospitals' need to rely on recruiting and training local people, despite historic low-wage structures, despite the large turnover rates characteristic of a young female labor supply—despite these and other difficulties and hurdles the hospitals and other health institutions have demonstrated a remarkable capacity to attract and retain ever larger numbers of allied health manpower so that today these nonprofessionals account for just under half of all the persons engaged in providing health services to the American people. If the record since the end of World War II can be interpreted in so favorable a light, what ground is there for concern about the future?

There are several untoward factors that cannot be ignored. The cost of medical care is rising steeply, principally in hospitals where wages and salaries account for about 60 percent of total expenditures. The only prospect of moderating this advance is through methods that could slow the rise in wage costs. The fact that more federal money is flowing into the financing of hospital care through Medicare and Medicaid, together with changes in legislative and administrative practices facilitating unionization, are likely to push in the opposite direction. The pressure for wage increases, especially for the lowly paid, will be intensified. So much on the cost side.

Consideration must also be given to the forces that continue to operate on the side of demand. The American public has taken at least halting steps in recent years to broaden the access to health services for the poor and the near poor. New experiments to deliver health services to the ghetto populations are under way. A large-scale expansion of nursing care for the aged is definitely planned. In addition to these pressures to meet the hitherto unmet demands for various types of health care of important groups in the population, the leadership in medicine continues to stress that real progress requires that quality gains go hand in hand with increases in the quantity of services to be provided. With allied health manpower often trained in makeshift programs, with many leaving employment a few years after being trained, with professional barriers to the orderly progression of those who acquire knowledge and experience, licensing requirements, and poor personnel management, the obstacles to quality improvement are as serious, if not more, than those standing in the way of meeting the quantitative manpower goals implicit in an expanding system of health care. It is against this background that the potentialities for public policy must be assessed.

A careful reading of the Greenfield–Brown book suggests that improvements in the recruitment, education and training, and utilization of allied health manpower can come about only through a variety of innovative actions at many different leverage points in the system of medical and health care.

To begin with recruitment. A field which attracts a disproportionate number of women, many of them young, will tend to have the following characteristics: a low wage scale, heavy turnover, excessive training costs, and relatively little accumulation of skill through experience. While some of these characteristics, such as a relatively low wage scale, are attractive to employers, it is not a pure gain especially in an industry which confronts the need for rapid growth. Moreover, if an industry cannot meet competitive wage standards, it runs the additional risk of not attracting the quality of workers who can absorb training and experience and readily be promoted.

A few experiments are under way on the East Coast, in the South, and in the West to attract into the civilian health industry former servicemen who were trained for and assigned to medical duties while on active service and who enjoyed their work and would be happy to continue in it if they could foresee a reasonable career ahead. Obvious social and personal gains would follow the building of such bridges. But recruitment is the easier part of the effort. The real challenge is to the hospitals and other health agencies which must open up meaningful career opportunities for those working at the lower levels of the hierarchy.[2]

The pressure of unionization which is slowly growing should contribute to the building of bridges between occupational levels. Among the most important demands that workers usually make is an expansion of opportunities to which they have access. Currently, the availability of federal training funds, particularly MDTA (Manpower Development and Training Act) funds, have made it easier for a few progressive unions and employers to design training programs aimed at the eventual promotion of workers from less-skilled to more-skilled jobs.

But obstacles remain to introducing mobility in the health manpower hierarchy for workers who begin at or near the bottom. At each rung of the ladder there are one or more organized groups whose principal aim has been to erect barriers aimed at reducing other workers' access. In most instances they have succeeded in gaining the approval of the state training authorities for their conditions and often they have further protected themselves by having their requirements approved by one of the principal health organizations, such as the American Medical Association or the American Hospital Association. Under these conditions they are in a powerful position to fend off encroachment.

It will require the cooperative efforts of many different groups to reduce barriers that have no justification other than to protect the position of those already ensconced. The demand for health care continues apace, and if the only foreseeable way of meeting this demand is through the rapid expansion of allied health manpower, the preconditions for some easing of restrictive arrangements may exist if hospitals and nursing homes join together with trade unions, medical societies, state licensing boards, and consumer groups to rewrite the laws and administrative practices, and if they move simultaneously and energetically to develop effective training and promotion policies which will open multiple career lines. It can be done but it surely will not be easy.

A second major thrust must be to improve the education

and training of allied health manpower. In recent years a beginning has been made to move beyond the confines of the individual hospital which in the past was the principal and sometimes the sole trainer of health personnel and to expand training through vocational education in high schools, in junior colleges, and in the newly established schools of allied health. These are important steps, and when these extensions have stressed a common core of much of the training, they have contributed to the eventual mobility of the manpower pool. Moreover, the transfer of much of the responsibility for didactic health training to the educational system should lead to a strengthening of the curriculum.

But once again we must beware of the difficulties that lie along this route. In the past, most state departments of health and education have had little to do with one another. Yet this new approach will require that they work in close harmony if the program is to succeed. Moreover, many young people who enter junior or senior college are likely to be pressed to take a broad liberal arts program together with their vocational or technical courses. In any case the collegiate environment encourages them to become more interested in acquiring a degree than in a salable skill. Finally, many, if not most, hospitals have provided training free of charge and some have even paid their trainees a modest sum, whereas in most junior and senior colleges students must pay tuition and fees. In shifting more and more training from the hospital to the educational system, care must be taken not to freeze out the many young people from low-income homes who have provided in the past, and must be expected to provide in the future, a significant proportion of all recruits to the health services industry. Liberal scholarship programs and expanded work-study arrangements might compensate for these untoward concomitants of a shift in the training sector.

In recent years the federal government, through the Allied Health Professions Personnel Training Act of 1966, has sought to contribute to the expansion of allied health manpower through appropriating modest sums for expanding training facilities, for the training of faculty, and for the support of experimental programs aimed at increasing the quantity and improving the quality of the total training effort. The current level of federal financing for these several purposes is about $15 million per annum. It is never safe to guess the future actions of Congress, but it appears unlikely that federal appropriations will be significantly increased in the foreseeable future when consideration is given to the present cautionary attitude toward all research and development spending, the priority position of physicians and nurses in commanding financial support, and the fact that in allied health manpower there are such large numbers of persons that any effort to single out their education for federal support would carry an implicit move to subsidize junior and senior college education on a large scale. Until Congress makes a major move in this direction, it is questionable whether it will take but modest additional steps to support directly the education and training of allied health manpower.

The federal effort consists of more than this single act.

At its last session (1968) Congress undertook a major national commitment to increase federal appropriations for vocational education. And while the health occupations account for a small percentage of all training, circa 5 percent, it is likely that they will expand rapidly.

Attention must also be directed to the MDTA, which was extended by overwhelming bipartisan support at the ninetieth session of Congress. Expenditure levels under this Act are at about half a billion dollars annually and about 20 percent of all training is in the health occupations. Clearly this is a sizable contribution.

Reference has been made to the constant and large-scale training in the health professions provided by the Armed Services and the prospects that exist if the civilian sector can introduce reforms which will enable it to use the ex-servicemen who have been trained and who served in medical assignments.

A comprehensive review of the potential contribution of the federal government would also include reference to the experimental community health centers under the Office of Economic Opportunity, the Regional Programs for Heart, Stroke, and Cancer, and the institutional and program efforts in mental health, vocational rehabilitation, public health, and care for veterans for which the federal government undertakes or finances the training of allied health manpower.

Nevertheless, the locus for action under our present distribution of responsibilities lies with state and local governments, which continue to have primary responsibility for the financing of education at the secondary and postsecondary levels. Whether the communities of the United States will be able to secure the numbers and the quality of allied health manpower they need to meet the steadily expanding demands for medical and health care will depend primarily on the capabilities of the existing health institutions to continue to train their own people, and whether state and local governments are willing and able to make public funds available to broaden and strengthen the training structure by bringing it increasingly under the rubric of the public educational system.

However, effective recruitment and utilization, as distinct from training, will continue to depend on the nongovernmental sector. The health services industry will be able to attract and retain the numbers and quality of allied health manpower it will need to meet its continuously expanding requirements only if the several leadership groups —hospitals, trade unions, professional organizations, consumers—recognize the need for additional change. No industry can respond effectively to the market unless it can attract the resources it requires.

The health services industry will continue to require large numbers of additional workers below the professional level. The challenge it faces is to modernize and rationalize its career structures so that the numbers it will require will be attracted into training and into employment.

❧ 12 ❧

Nursing Realities

There may be an advantage to an outsider's look at a discipline, an occupation, or a professional group, since distance often lends perspective. This may be particularly apposite in a look at the labor market where no group stands alone. The student of manpower may see linkages which the members of a particular group do not see although they are affected by them.

The supply of nurses has been fairly responsive to the increasing demand despite complaints of continuing shortages.[1] There are more nurses engaged in nursing today; there are more different kinds of people involved in nursing service than we would have thought possible two decades ago. The ratio of nurses to the population has gone up, not down.[2]

The assumption that there is a nursing shortage is wrong on two counts. First, there cannot be a "shortage" that lasts over twenty years. There can be a shortage for a short time, but in an open society, an open economy, a "shortage" cannot continue indefinitely. Second, since the ratio of nurses to the population has increased, what does a shortage of nurses mean? Certainly not every hospital in every region has all the nursing personnel that it would like to employ for the amount of money that it is able or willing to pay. Using this criterion, however, we are short of a great many things in this country. We are short of good professors at our universities, we are short of beautiful actresses in Hollywood, we are short of good politicians in Washington. But little meaning can attach to the statement that the nursing profession is characterized by acute shortages. What has happened, of course, is that although more and more women have gone into nursing, the American consumer has had the means to pay for still more health services, including nursing services.

There is a remote possibility—and it may not be so remote—that a permanent gap will develop between the amount of nursing care that the American people desire and require and the number of younger and older women who will be willing to enter and remain in the field at present and prospective levels of salaries and other appurtenances. In that event we may be forced to take a leaf from the Japanese, who have an unique pattern for coping with this problem. In Japan the family moves into the hospital and cooks for and nurses the patient. If our situation gets very tight, we may still come to that. Each of the three times my wife was delivered in a good New York hospital, I served as an ad hoc nurse and kept count of the frequency of her labor pains!

A Backward Look

One way to get a perspective on where we are now and

on where we are likely to go in the future is to take a retrospective view of the changes that have occurred since the end of World War II.

Although they were slow in coming, there have been major corrections in the market place with regard to wages and working conditions. It took considerable time for the improvements to be introduced but they have been commendable.

In the late 1940s married women were not welcome in the field of nursing, surely not for part-time employment. But reality intruded and the profession adjusted.

On the educational front, many approved and nonapproved hospital schools of nursing have closed and more will follow suit.[3] In the past two decades the federal government has become a significant factor, first in underwriting graduate education for nurses and more recently in financing basic nursing education. This has been a major change. There has been a steady, if not spectacular, increase in college-trained nurses.[4]

The professional nursing associations have struggled during the past two decades to find satisfactory solutions to the relationships that should exist among nurses with different levels of training—baccalaureate degree, three-year diploma course, two-year associate degree, one-year practical nurse diploma, three-months nurse's aide training—and the preferred patterns of nurse utilization in and out of hospitals.[5]

Uncertainty and confusion, however, continue to characterize these relationships as a result of the inherent difficulties of correlating new patterns of training with new approaches to utilization. Despite strong leadership, professional organizations cannot move readily toward new goals and objectives if their members see a possible threat to their livelihood.

These then have been the major changes in the nursing profession. Supply has increased in response to demand. Changes on the educational front have come more slowly. Utilization patterns continue in disarray. Wages and working conditions have improved, particularly recently. The leadership still has serious problems to contend with because of splits among the members.

Current Realities

So much for the past. Where does nursing stand today? First, planning for the nursing profession must start from the premise that diploma nurses will remain the dominant group for many years to come. This is the only possible deduction based on the laws of arithmetic.

The second simple fact of life is that nursing education still is in a vulnerable position because it remains largely outside of the mainstream of American educational effort. Many diploma schools are closing because of financial difficulties. On the other hand, several major private universities have abandoned undergraduate baccalaureate programs for nurses—among other reasons because of excessive costs. The most favorable trend is the growth of the Associate programs, which continue to multiply rapidly.[6] Such programs have the advantage of being publicly financed.

The fact that some diploma schools and baccalaureate schools charge $1,000 or more for tuition at a time when the profession is anxiously seeking to attract more students underscores the unsatisfactory state of nursing education. No effective solution is likely to be found outside of transferring most of the responsibility for nursing education to the public purse.

Wages and working conditions will continue to improve, but this will not be an unmixed boon to all. As the salary of the diploma nurse, the baccalaureate nurse, and the graduate nurse is raised still higher, every purchaser—hospital administrators, clinic administrators, nursing-home administrators—will seek protection in the principle of substitution. Each will try to get his job done by using less-expensive personnel. This is the inevitable response of management whenever wages are raised. Employers always look for more economical ways of covering their personnel needs and they redouble their efforts when their wage costs rise steeply.

There are additional pressures for administrators to move in this direction. An unpublished report of a large hospital in a mid-Atlantic state recently analyzed 92 nursing functions in terms of whether it was preferable to have a diploma nurse, a practical nurse, or nurse's aide perform them and compared the results with the actual assignment of personnel to these functions. The study found that in the opinion of the professional members of the staff, about 25 percent of the functions should have been performed by a diploma or practical nurse, and 75 percent could have been performed by aides. But the actual educational background was inverted: 75 percent were diploma nurses or practical nurses, and 25 percent were aides. This study suggests the continuing difficulties of developing a balance between the output of the schools and the ways in which hospital and other administrators use and prefer to use the various categories of nursing personnel available to them.

There will inevitably continue to be tensions among competing groups of trained personnel. A nurse with a newly acquired baccalaureate obviously does not have as much experience as a practical nurse with ten years on the floor. But she may receive the same or even a higher salary. The variability in educational background and specialized training among diploma nurses, practical nurses, and nurse's aides creates difficulties in assigning them as well as in rewarding them. The likelihood is that no administrator can satisfy all of these groups; often he satisfies none of them. While education is important, experience contributes greatly to the skill of a nurse, as it does to every other professional. Experience is tremendously important and it is not acquired by certification. Certification can make only an initial discrimination.

There is, moreover, little possibility that the professional nurse associations will be able to draw definite boundaries between themselves and other less-trained groups. And there is even less prospect of their maintaining whatever boundaries they do establish. These boundaries differ among states, among cities, even among institutions within the same city. They cannot be fixed once and for all time; there are too many forces operating to unsettle them.

The Options Nurses Face

The medical scene is being rapidly transformed. Health care in the United States is today a $56 billion industry, and there are responsible forecasts that by 1975 total expenditures will exceed a $100 billion or approximate 10 percent of the GNP. An industry of such scale cannot hope to remain the private province of a small number of professional groups. It impinges with too much force on too many different sectors of the society. Most importantly it must be responsive to those who pay the bill—consumer, insurance carriers, government. Because of rapidly rising costs, the American consumer will be interested in and will insist upon greater economies in the delivery of health care services. These are some of the options that nurses confront.

They can devote themselves to improving the existing confused patterns of training and utilization.

They can opt in favor of a higher degree of clinical competence with corresponding changes in duties.

They can make a bid for broader administrative responsibilities in hospitals and nursing homes.

To the outsider looking in, it appears that most of the efforts and energies of the leadership have been directed since the end of World War II to the first option.

There have been a plethora of studies focused on developing more effective patterns of utilization to insure that the most highly trained nurses do not undertake tasks that could just as well be performed by more modestly trained

members of the team. But, as has been noted, variability
in training patterns, in manpower availabilities, and in
wage and salary levels have made it not only difficult but
impossible for the profession to establish optimal patterns
of staffing. There is no reason to believe that additional
efforts along these lines will prove more satisfactory. Frustration is built into the situation.

What are the prospects with respect to the second option
which sees the nurse developing a high level of clinical
competence? The challenge here is whether, with the help
of the public that desires to see medical costs controlled,
nurses can persuade the medical profession to restudy their
work patterns and make suitable adjustments. We know
that much of the work that a pediatrician, an allergist, a
surgeon performs in his office could be done very satisfac-
torily by a trained nurse. The same holds for many aspects
of obstetrical and gynecological care. There is also much
room for the transfer of responsibilities from physicians to
nurses in the care of various groups of chronic patients,
particularly those who are treated at home or in a clinic.
In addition, much work can be shifted from the physician
to the nurse within the hospital—in the operating room,
the delivery room, the receiving room, and in various diagnostic and therapeutic stations.

To meet such increased responsibilities, nurses would of
course require additional training in various clinical specialties. But if a way could be found to assure that the
medical dollar were more equitably distributed between
the physician and the nurse to take account of such shifts,

many nurses would undoubtedly be willing to take the additional training. If this could be accomplished, everybody would be better off—the physician, the nurse, and the patient.

Progress along these lines would necessitate alterations in the present haphazard system of training nurses for clinical specialties. The leadership of the nursing profession would have to take the lead to persuade more universities and medical centers to provide effective instruction at both undergraduate and graduate levels aimed at clinical specialization, and the appropriate nursing associations would have to take steps toward the certification of such clinical specialists.

Another arena of expanding opportunities for nurses relates to the management of hospitals and nursing homes. One reason that hospital costs are so high and are going steadily higher is that a hospital is not really managed. It is unlikely that the American public will tolerate hospital costs of $100 and more per day without insisting upon much tighter management. The classic British pattern, for example, is one in which the nurse-matron has control over all patient-related personnel except the physician. It is questionable whether the nursing profession in the United States could at this late date succeed in securing such authority even if they made a bid for it.

A more likely development is that nurses will increasingly go after managerial positions in nursing homes. Nurses have for a long time managed small hospitals and nursing homes. The advent of Medicare and Medicaid foreshadows a rapid expansion in less intensive medical care facilities. If more nurses at both undergraduate and graduate level sought training in finance, management, and personnel they would be able to compete for these highly attractive positions. The opportunity is there.

From Confusion to Clarification

For the last two decades much of the effort of the nursing profession has gone into seeking order out of the confusion in which nursing services are provided in the hospital. The leaders have sought to specify what type of nurse should do what, to which patient, under what conditions. But a reading of the past reveals that the situation got beyond the control of the nursing profession. The hospital administrator who had to find staff to cover his floors, the physician who needed help in caring for his patient, and the patient who had to pay the bill, were more potent in determining the emerging patterns than were the leaders of the nursing profession. This was true in the past and it will be true in the future.

There is one other basic task that the leadership entered upon many years ago to which it should continue to devote time and effort. No matter which option the profession prefers—and the odds are good that all these options should be open to women with different abilities and desires—there is need to speed the transfer of responsibility for nursing education from the hospital to the educational system. Without a sound educational and training structure—

properly staffed and financed—little improvement can be achieved. But assuming that the present trends in this direction are accelerated, the leadership will still face many challenges.

It must find ways of reducing the training time required for bedside nursing in a supervised environment of hospital and nursing home. Unless it can break through its own organizational constraints and give the public an honest answer, it will not be able to talk with authority and its influence will be further diminished.

It must explore in cooperation with the leaders of the medical profession, the faculties of medical schools, and the staffs of the principal teaching hospitals, what changes are required and how they can be speeded to open up new and meaningful careers for clinical nurse specialists and then take steps to arrange suitable training and methods of certification.

Finally it must appraise realistically what its competitive advantages and limitations are with respect to making a bid for filling more administrative positions. It may be too late for the nurse to take back from the hospital administrator and his staff responsibility for control over all nonprofessional ancillary personnel. But if nurses were properly trained, that is, if they had, in addition to basic nurse training and ward experience, graduate courses in management and personnel, they might still be able to compete for such critically important positions. It is surely not too late for them—but it soon may be—to compete for positions as administrators of nursing homes.

The nursing profession has been living with disorder

for a long time. It is a difficult environment in which to
work, but it would be sensible for both the leadership and
the membership to realize that the disorder is likely to persist for a long time to come. New opportunities, however,
are looming on the horizon. The task of the leadership is
to turn its back on mirages and to grapple with reality.

❧13❧
Clinical Laboratory Personnel

There are two views of modern medicine. One sees health care as the epitome of modern science in which the full panoply of new theories and esoteric techniques is used in diagnosing and treating the patient. The back-up of open-heart and transplant surgery with extensive electronic monitoring illustrates this view. The other is an older, less dramatic assessment of contemporary medicine; while acknowledging that the wonders of science have taken over at the margin, this view sees most people who need, seek, and obtain treatment as receiving less dramatic diagnosis and therapy.

One wise diagnostician pointed out some years ago the differences between his predecessors, who had made their reputation on brilliant hunches and insights, and the run-of-the-mill physician of today. If the latter is conscientious, he will be able with the help of the laboratory to make the right diagnosis in 95 percent of the illnesses presented to him. He does not need to be inspired to practice good medicine if he is willing to check himself by judicious use of the laboratory.

It is the laboratory that has helped to turn medicine from art into science. Consequently, the proper staffing and operating of laboratories lie at the center of good medicine. But, as the following analysis will seek to make clear, there are many difficulties in the path of accomplishing these two critical objectives.

Structure and Trends

In looking closely at the clinical laboratory, particularly from the point of view of manpower, one can see in microcosm the range of complex forces operating on the health services industry that simultaneously make it possible for the industry to respond to new challenges and opportunities while confronting new barriers as it seeks to adapt to change.

Although we talk of the health services industry as a homogeneous segment of the economy, it is hardly that. With regard to clinical laboratories, we must distinguish at least the following varieties. First are those located in hospitals, concerned principally with the diagnosis and treatment of inpatients but which often also provide services for the staff members who find it convenient to use the hospital laboratory in their private practice. Second, there are laboratories of departments of public health which tend to specialize in tests related to their principal charge of monitoring various infectious and contagious diseases and to test for certain environmental hazards. Third, there are commercial laboratories, run for profit, which provide support for the private practitioner as well as for many smaller and some large hospitals which prefer to use these services rather than expand the range of their own laboratory services.

With improved air transportation and the greater sophistication required for some of the difficult new testing procedures, major medical centers on the East Coast send a certain type of work to a highly specialized laboratory in the Los Angeles area, secure in the knowledge that the results will be back in three to four days and, more important, that they will be right. Since the man-machine confrontation required for maximum accuracy is difficult to achieve with respect to these clinical tests, the laboratory in Los Angeles now serves the national market.

Although there are no firm figures about the number of laboratories, the tests which they perform, the manpower they use, and the reliability of their work, the following overview was pieced together from existing reports; it may not be badly askew. According to reports of the National Communicable Diseases Center and the American Hospital Association, it appears that most hospitals have a clinical laboratory, which means that there are approximately 7,000 hospital-based laboratories. It is estimated that state and local public health departments together have a total of 400, and that there are about 6,000 independent, commercially operated laboratories. In addition, many physicians do some laboratory work in their offices; the number may total 40,000.[1]

As to work load, a rough estimate comes to half a billion tests annually. More important the output has been rising at a rate of about 15 percent per annum, which means a doubling every five years. The experts believe that the rate of increase will be maintained in the years ahead in response to a variety of pressures that tend to reinforce each other. Automation of existing laboratories is creating a large new capacity, which will invite use. Physicians are increasingly trained in "scientific medicine," which means that they tend to rely more and more on the laboratory for support. The passage of Medicare and Medicaid has lowered the restraints on many physicians who had previously hesitated to prescribe additional procedures for low-income patients. Finally, advances in medicine itself are constantly adding to the power of diagnostic tools. The physician is able, especially when baffled, to pursue leads that formerly were not available to him.

There are certain other characteristics of clinical laboratory work within the larger rubric of medical services that should be put in place before the focus is shifted to the manpower dimension. The work load tends to be differentiated between a limited number of basic tests and a large number of specialized tests. It has been estimated that of the chemistry tests now available, "some 20 tests comprise 80 percent of the daily chemistry work load." The great potential of automation lies in the arena where there is large volume and where the technology can be adapted. Dr. John Knowles, of Massachusetts General Hospital, reported recently that the costs of certain routine tests had been reduced to a point where the paper work to bill the patient accounted for more than the cost of the test. But before we jump to the conclusion that in the near future hospitals are likely to absorb routine laboratory tests as part of their per diem costs, we must note that many of them have charged in excess of their costs for years. It was one way of balancing their books, although the ratio of the costs of clinical laboratory tests to total expenses has been about 5 to 10 percent.

The gains from potential automation affect not only costs but quality. While poor work can be done under automated procedures—failure to check limits and to use quality control methods are among the common failings—in general the machine, under proper supervision, is more reliable than a man without it.

A large volume of routine tests done with increasing automation points clearly in the direction of more centralized laboratories in large population centers. While large hospitals will not quickly slough off their clinical laboratories because they want to maintain an in-house capability to cope with complex tests and to do them quickly, the trend appears to be in the direction of large, increasingly automated laboratories. It is likely that these will be more and more in the private sector of the economy and that various corporate enterprises with related expertise may soon enter the field in large numbers. While some leaders of the medical profession, particularly those who stand to lose by this potential competition, will probably fight a rear-guard action, the early court decisions suggest that their opposition will not succeed.

As laboratory services become more sophisticated, we will probably see an expansion of reference laboratories geared to perform specialized and complex tests. These are likely to serve a whole region, and some the entire country.

Another development will be the expansion of bedside units equipped to monitor critical responses of the body. Most of these will be located in intensive care units and in emergency rooms.

That leaves the small laboratory which must support the small hospital in less-populated areas as well as local practitioners and specialists who need tests made on their ambulatory patients. We know from a recent Minnesota study of the great difficulties in staffing and operating these small laboratories.

A word about supervision and control of clinical laboratory work will complete this brief discussion of structure and trends. As with much of medical care, control is more conspicuous by its absence than by its presence. Good teaching hospitals seek to run good clinical laboratories, and most of them reach a satisfactory level of performance most of the time. Laboratories in small hospitals and many of those under commercial auspices, however, are less satisfactory. A series of studies conducted in the 1950s revealed unsatisfactory test results, 25, 33, and 50 percent of the time.

States have varied in their efforts to establish and enforce standards but, with the passage of Medicare, the federal government established criteria for independent laboratories and thus helped to precipitate the problem of quality control. Nevertheless, it is a problem: for years one conscientious internist in New York City has been sending his materials to two laboratories since he does not feel he can trust either!

The performance of a laboratory is a function of its ability to attract and to supervise personnel. As in so many other aspects of medical care, personnel is the critical element.

The Manpower Picture

A first overview of the manpower scene can be obtained from a listing of the different types of persons who are employed. In hospital laboratories, pathologists are usually in charge, especially in the large hospitals, since they alone are permitted to diagnose on the basis of test results. All others, at least in theory, are constrained to report their findings to a physician, who then must make the interpretation.

Next come the biochemists, microbiologists, chemists— some with a Ph.D. or Doctor of Science, more with a master's degree—who may be in charge of a specialized laboratory in a large medical center under the overall direction of the pathologist, or who may independently be in charge of a laboratory in a smaller hospital or one that operates commercially. College graduates with a major in chemistry, biology, biochemistry are employed in large numbers and usually function as medical technologists in general or specialized laboratories.

Following in descending order are:

Medical technologists who have been certified by the American Society of Clinical Pathologists (ASCP) on the basis of at least three years of college and one year of clini-

cal training in an accredited program. The total number
of registered MT (ASCP) in 1967 was slightly over 44,000,
up from 22,000 in eleven years.

Individuals with some or no college education, who have
been school-trained (usually under commercial auspices)
hospital-trained, or trained on the job in nonprofit, governmental, or commercial laboratories and who perform
the work of a medical technologist.

Cytotechnologists—specialists in cancer tests—who have
had two years of college plus one year of training in an
approved program. There are now about 2,000 certified
cytotechnologists.

Closely related are the histologic technicians (about
3,100), high-school graduates with one year of supervised
training, who specialize in screening cancer cells and in
cutting and straining body tissue for examination. There
are also those who perform these tasks who have not been
trained in accredited programs.

Laboratory assistants, who help technologists and technicians by performing simple tests. Most of them have gone
through unaccredited programs or have been trained on
the job.

Helpers and bottle washers with no training.

There is no reliable count of all who are employed in
clinical laboratory services; two recent estimates set the
figure between 85,000 and 100,000. Within this total there
is a wide spread among qualifications, both general and
specific, as well as a marked variability in how people have
been trained. Moreover, there is substantial substituta-

bility among various levels of personnel. If better educated and better trained men or women cannot be employed because they are not available or the salary they demand is beyond what has been budgeted, the head of the laboratory seeks to utilize those who have less education and training but who he believes will be able to handle the assignment.

As in almost every field within the medical structure, the leadership has attempted to establish educational and training standards for certification and employment. The pathologists and the medical technologists have cooperated for many years to this end and they have elicited the support of the Council on Medical Education of the American Medical Association. Since the hospital and scientific medicine have become ever more important in recent years, the number of AMA Accredited Schools of Medical Technology increased from under 600 in 1955 to about 800 in 1967. This was accompanied by an increase of about 80 percent in enrollment and in graduates.

However recent experience has not been a straightforward expansion under the impetus and direction of the establishment. Several parallel trends should be noted. Commercial schools—except in California, which established the requirements of a college degree, postgraduate laboratory apprenticeship, and a stiff examination for a medical technologist's license—continue to exist and some flourish in helping to meet a strong local demand. Programs financed by the federal government under the Manpower Development and Training Act have trained significant numbers of medical technicians and other laboratory personnel. There has been a spectacular increase in junior colleges which, in search of occupational programs, have begun to direct their attention to preparing students for the health services industry, including positions in clinical laboratories. A few localities now pay particular attention to the considerable number of servicemen who, while on active duty are trained for and assigned to clinical laboratories; some of these men desire to follow this career upon their return to civilian life. Efforts have been intensified to identify these young men, provide them with refresher and up-grading opportunities, and to locate desirable assignments for them.

In each of these programs—commercial schools, MDTA programs, junior colleges, and special programs for veterans—pulls are being exerted against the trend in which pathologists and the MT (ASCP) are striving to raise standards and to control access to employment and promotion.

There is one development, the establishment of Colleges of Allied Health Professions, in which Florida has taken the lead, where the effort is to speed the "professionalization" of medical supporting staff by bringing more of it within the rubric of colleges and universities, to improve its quality by stress on a core curriculum, and to improve career opportunities by facilitating mobility. It is too early to tell whether and how fast this new effort will spread. But since it is directed to important objectives, it will probably grow, if not as rapidly as its proponents originally anticipated.

Pulls and Counter-Pulls

The conventional view is that clinical laboratory personnel are in short supply as are personnel in other health areas and that, unless special efforts are made, these shortages are likely to worsen as the demand for care continues to expand. A 1966 survey of personnel needs in hospitals reported a shortage of medical technologists of approximately 7.5 percent and of laboratory assistants of almost 5 percent.

The reported vacancy rate for clinical laboratory technologists in California at the beginning of 1967 was estimated at 8 percent, the lowest it had been in fifteen years. Since California has such high standards for licensing and since it must replace annually about 15 percent of its total supply because of attrition, it is not the size but the smallness of the gap between supply and demand that is impressive.

An incisive assessment of the manpower scene, present and future, must take at least the following variables into account: the characteristics of the persons attached to the field, training capacity, wages and working conditions, turnover, career opportunities, and of course the future demand for services.

In light of the unknowns which will be introduced by automation and the advances of medical science, it is indeed difficult to foretell the shape of future demand. One careful student of the subject has calculated that while the total demand for medical manpower will increase by

approximately one-third during the decade 1965-75, the
increase in demand for medical laboratory personnel is
likely to be twice as large. But there are questions about
whether this differentially more rapid rate of expansion
of laboratory manpower will in fact occur. The study an-
ticipates that the effects of automation will continue to
be felt and that in general they will reduce the demand
for manpower.

The next question is whether compensating factors, such
as the multiplication of multiphasic screening, will lead
to an enhanced demand for manpower despite an improved
technology. Estimates suggest that there will soon be units
with the capacity to work with large groups at a cost of
between $15-$30 per patient, including amortization of
equipment within five years and including fees paid to
physicians. Until the data banks now being accumulated
by Kaiser-Permanente and the Public Health Service have
been analyzed and evaluated, it will be difficult to foretell the potentiality of multiphasic screening. But one outcome is certain: If the trials prove that this approach holds
the promise of early detection of disease among a significant proportion of those screened, it will probably undergo
rapid expansion.

Further evidence of the uncertain future of laboratories
is found in the *Annual Report for 1966-67* of the National
Committee for Careers in Medical Technology. The report appraised the period ahead: "Just what technological
change, automation, data processing, centralization, and
regionalization will do . . . is still a matter of conjecture
as is the effect of the new specialists in medical engineering

and electronics as well as the new classes of laboratory assistants."

There was general agreement, however, among the members of the Manpower Conference in Washington in October, 1967, that there is sufficient thrust to the trend toward automation that laboratories will increasingly require specialists with sophisticated training in computer skills who will henceforth play an ever-larger role in organizing and directing the laboratories' work. But even this consensus about the direction of new manpower needs left several questions unanswered: how these specialists can best be trained, the amount of general education they should have, their relation to other personnel in the laboratory, particularly those with more medical and less technical competence.

The uncertainty of future demand, both with regard to general and specific level, requires caution in developing manpower projections for the future. But the direction of future change can be delineated although the details cannot be filled in.

With regard to supply and utilization of manpower, there are some current problem areas which might cast a shadow ahead. The first is that a recent survey of college-trained medical technologists working in hospitals showed that there are approximately 3 women for every 1 man. If hospital personnel with less education and training were included, the ratio might well be 7 women to 1 man. Another recent survey disclosed that the dropout rate among students during their fourth year of clinical training was under 5 percent. The report mistakenly compared this

rate with an attrition rate of 33 percent among nurses during their three years of study. Even when corrected, this
comparison shows a low attrition rate for medical technology students.

A careful review of the medical manpower situation in
Minnesota concluded that "in our state as elsewhere, the
average female medical technologist has an active 'half-
life' of two years. Few return to laboratory work after
bearing their first child." While these conclusions about
Minnesota cannot be fully reconciled with the finding that
California has an annual turnover rate of approximately
15 percent or that 40 percent of all who are licensed in
California are inactive, they do point in the same direction
of high attrition rates after the trainees have been qualified
and begin to work.

A fuller understanding of job-turnover rates requires
that we consider, in addition to the sex and age of the personnel—young women of marriageable age who comprise
the majority of medical technologists are the most likely
to withdraw from the labor market—the wage and career
progression opportunities which are likely to exercise a
strong influence on the shape of original recruitment and
later retention.

Before looking more closely at these critically important
factors we must recall that medical technology is "a young
profession with nearly three-fourths of its members having
less than 10 years experience." A large questionnaire survey of certified medical technologists revealed that three-
quarters were less than 39 years old and 42 percent were
less than 30. (In this sample only 11 percent were male!)

Because of unusually dynamic growth and somewhat skewed distribution, we must be especially cautious in making projections based on past experience.

As part of this questionnaire, a salary survey in 1967 (1966 data) based on replies from 70 percent of all those on the Registry revealed the following interesting facts about the structure: the median salary was $6,144, up 18 percent from the 1962 level. One in almost 4 technicians earns between $7,200 and $7,800 and 1 in 6 earns more than $7,800. Since the period after 1966 has probably seen a comparable rise, this would bring the median salary at the end of 1969 to about $7,000.

Other interesting findings are the following: there is a variation of about $1,000 between the salaries of persons employed in hospitals and those in industry in favor of the latter. Those who had just started to work averaged about $5,500, while those who had been in the field for ten to twenty years earned an average of less than $6,900— a narrow range indeed. The same narrow spread existed among personnel with different functions: while the staff technologist earned on the average $5,800, the section head received less than $6,500 and the chief medical technologist only $6,900. There was less than a $200 spread in annual earnings among those with no degree, those with a junior college degree, and those with a baccalaureate. Moreover only $150 separated those with a doctorate from those with a master's degree. The only significant differential was found between those who had acquired a master's degree and those with a baccalaureate: here the spread came to $1,600.

As one might have anticipated from general knowledge of geographic differentials, these loomed large. The spread between California and Maine was of the order of 45 percent; the differences among large cities was even larger; the salary level in Los Angeles was about 52 percent above that of Pittsburgh.

These data raise a series of interesting questions. While the leadership has been pressing to raise educational requirements to assure that more clinical laboratory personnel are trained at least to the level of the baccalaureate, the salary data give no evidence that such an investment will be rewarded—unless of course the individual is able and willing to go on to acquire a master's degree. But other evidence indicates that many graduate institutions will not admit individuals who have acquired their baccalaureate in medical technology! To add to the difficulties, the number of schools which provide graduate instruction in medical technology are relatively limited, and fellowship aid for people in this field is relatively scarce. Moreover, the entire salary scale is compressed. A person can look forward to small and few increments after a decade in the field, even if he is promoted into the top job.

In sum, the present salary and career structure is unattractive to men. Moreover, several rungs on the career ladder are missing. It is difficult to move from one level of work to another and even if one succeeds, rewards are frequently so small as to be insignificant. In light of the large numbers of women who withdraw after a few years in the field, attention should be directed to developing the reentry routes. While the leadership is aware that the recruitment and retention of competent personnel present difficulties, there are many areas in which they cannot by themselves introduce relevant reforms. They can try to modify training programs and certification procedures. But it is only the pressures of the market place and new entrepreneurial structures that are likely to modify radically salary levels and career opportunities. These have been operating to some extent in the recent past; the major remaining uncertainty is whether private commercial laboratories, under the stimulus of the new technology and opportunities for volume work, will take the lead and radically restructure the personnel system.

If, as appears likely, this happens, it would imply that laboratories will shift from a preoccupation with the educational qualifications of the staff to a concern with the quality of the output. This would clearly be a move forward. There is, in addition, the prospect that changes in commercial laboratories will be the harbinger of changes in the provision of medical services. These will occur only under the combined influence of new entrepreneurial structures, more rationalized systems of combining men and machines, and more emphasis on the quality of the output than on the educational qualifications of the manpower. The prospective changes in commercial laboratories may be a good omen of things to come.

❧14❧
Social Workers

Many professionals are dismayed to realize that the problems with which they have been struggling are not specific to their field but can be duplicated in many other fields. As a result of his specialized education and training, the professional is inclined to believe that his work is unique. And it may well be. Too often he forgets that before one becomes a specialist he is a member of a larger undifferentiated student and work body.

A large number of fields therefore compete for the same limited manpower pool. Social work is but one of many career options available to the same group of people. Second, recruitment is but one small aspect of a manpower program. Employee retention is no less essential for the vitality of an organization and the successful implementation of its program. In social work, as in many related fields such as teaching and nursing, this point is frequently overlooked.

A third point relates to the differential work patterns of men and women and their implications for social work. Other things being equal, the more women, especially young women, employed in a field, the higher the attrition rate. French's follow-up studies of social workers found a loss of full-time young women workers during the seven-year period, 1957-64, of some 60 percent. By any standards, such an attrition rate is excessive. Moreover, a field which depends on a female labor force must have particular sensitivity to the reentry problems of mature women who wish to return to work.

A related fact is that most women marry, and once they marry their flexibility and mobility with respect to both education and training and employment is considerably reduced. These factors can be ignored only at a serious cost not only to the women themselves but also to employers who must depend on women for some or, as in the case of social work, most of their staff.

Economic considerations are also fundamental to realistic manpower planning. There is a general rule that all employers—private, governmental, nonprofit—seek the least expensive manpower with which they can accomplish their work, and even the most sincere commitment to professional standards is heavily counterbalanced by budgetary constraints. Effectiveness and economy are closely related, and it is incumbent upon every employer to extend his budget as far as possible in an effort to fulfill his program. By the same token, every professional group operates more or less like a union which seeks to limit entrance and to raise salaries. Modified somewhat by the traditions of professional practice, employers and employees behave according to the rule of the labor market.

Social welfare planning often reflects a failure to differentiate between need and demand. *Closing the Gap*, a recent HEW report, states that in 1970 there will be 100,000 vacancies for professionally trained social workers. Consider what that means in terms of money. Although Congress has recently been quite liberal in expanding health and welfare programs, it is not likely to vote funds of this magnitude for social work staff. So while the leadership is properly concerned with need, it would be an act of realism to consider demand, which is need plus the money to cover the need.

The next point has the quality of a paradox. There is a widespread assumption that in a dynamic society and economy, all systems become progressively more complicated and, therefore, more professionally trained people are needed. In brief, the demand for skill moves in only one direction—up. If that be the case, where are the benefits of greater affluence and more education? Logically, the opposite should occur. One would expect that if more and more individuals complete high school, more and more go on to college, more and more complete college, this "nation of better-educated Americans" could function with somewhat less social service. In some respects that is true. For example, one of the most important gains in pediatrics since World War II had nothing to do with scientific advances but resulted from Dr. Spock's book, which most American mothers were able to read and apply. Widespread literacy and low-cost distribution enabled Dr. Spock to make a greater contribution to the health of American children than might have occurred if 10,000 additional pediatricians had entered private practice. Essential revisions of need in response to such developments are rarely noted by professional or social action groups who try to influence Con-

gress to appropriate additional funds for expanding the
supply of professional manpower.

The field of engineering is another case in point. We
constantly hear that the country needs more engineers.
However, little note is taken of the fact that the computer
has eliminated perhaps as much as 40 percent of routine
engineering work. Detailed calculations, which a generation ago occupied most young engineers, are no longer
done by hand. Thus, progress may often be reflected in a
reduction in demand for manpower as well as in an increase
in demand.

Finally, we must question the basic assumption, common
to all professions, that more and more formal education is
the key to competence. Our national commitment to education notwithstanding, there is no predictable yield in
terms of superior job performance from additional study.
The relationship between work proficiency and academic
achievement depends upon how specific requirements are
related to specific tasks. It is a fallacy to rely exclusively
upon education as a standard for work assignment. Sometimes there is no alternative. In developing countries
where performance standards do not exist, education often
is the only clue to a person's fitness for a task. But in a
sophisticated society, there must be independent, specific
criteria for assessing performance and potential. For many
years the Armed Services sought to estimate military effectiveness solely on the basis of an AFQT score. Eventually
they devised additional tests to improve their screening.
While it would be wrong to deny the relevance of educational achievement, general manpower experience has

demonstrated that it is not the *sine qua non* of satisfactory performance.

What is the applicability of these general perspectives on manpower to social work? A good way to proceed is to appraise critically the HEW document *Closing the Gap*, which is the most comprehensive as well as the most recent document on social welfare manpower.[1]

The first recommendation of the report calls for a radical expansion of the schools of social work, with the goal of tripling student enrollment, especially in metropolitan centers. Ambitious as this program is, its implementation would still fail to satisfy the requirements for additional professionals stipulated elsewhere in the report. The question has been raised earlier how realistic these requirements are in terms of the market; nevertheless, the proposed solution would still fall short of need.

A more serious question is how effective the manpower yield of such a large-scale educational expansion would be in meeting the nation's actual need for service. *Closing the Gap* emphasizes the distributional problems: social services are most acutely lacking in areas of the country where no schools of social work exist. The location of new schools in metropolitan centers is likely to exacerbate, rather than to correct, this maldistribution. In addition, there is little evidence of the availability of "human resources"—faculty or potential students—needed to expand the schools. Capital requirements are another bottleneck, although funds can usually be more readily mobilized than people.

The program proposes two classes of social work manpower: those who have acquired master's degrees from

graduate schools of social work, and those with bacca-
laureates who have completed an undergraduate major in
social work. Unfortunately, the document leaves unclari-
fied the logic for this sharp distinction. The superiority of
two years of graduate social work training over a competent
four-year college course, including two years of a major in
social work, is not self-evident. Presumably, graduate education is more effective than undergraduate instruction. In
addition, there is ambiguity in the stated goals of undergraduate training: is it to prepare students for graduate
schools of social work and at the same time prepare them
for work?

Such a rigid distinction between bachelor's and master's
degrees poses utilization problems for the conscientious administrator. How is he to resolve the frequent promotion
dilemma—in favor of the individual with advanced training or the bright worker with only an undergraduate degree? How will this affect incentives for excellence and
devotion to the job, and ultimately the quality and effectiveness of the organization?

A third recommendation relates to recruitment which,
it is suggested, would be stimulated by the availability of
additional funds. As indicated earlier, recruitment is generally overemphasized as a solution to basic manpower
problems that beset a field: when salaries, working conditions, and relationships to other groups cause difficulties,
people look to recruitment to get around them. Recruitment may be a valid concern, but it seldom holds the solution to most manpower problems.

What about the recommended educational loans with

"forgiveness" provisions to those who pursue a career in the field? Once this device is adopted, should it not be extended to everyone who borrows money to go to college? It is questionable whether this particular type of "come-on," first offered to teachers, later to social workers, and still later, to other groups, is a sound way to proceed. Moreover, it is not clear that it will accomplish much. If recruitment is really a problem, it would be advisable to consider ways of attracting into the field those who are not applying primarily because money is a barrier. In one sense, recruitment is like competitive advertising: in a tight labor market it may be necessary to exploit it in order to maintain one's position, but it will probably not provide a basic solution.

The fourth recommendation is directed at improved retention by the twin expedients of admitting workers with a B.A. into the professional organizations and supporting their eligibility for state licensure. Liberalization of admission requirements will effectively augment the membership lists and the revenues of the professional societies, and it will enhance the status of the newly recognized workers, even if they are not given full membership. However, organizational strength and influence will be served best by a single membership category: consider the AMA, which does not distinguish between the general practitioner who has completed only an internship and the neurosurgeon who has had at least five years of residency training.

The status and protection provided the profession by licensing must also be viewed with caution. Although widely used to control manpower, its efficacy is limited.

Even psychiatrists, who belong to one of the most protected fraternities in the United States, the medical profession, have not gained much. Consider: if the number of people seeking help significantly exceeds the number of licensed practitioners, those in need will secure the services they require elsewhere—regardless of license. One has only to read the report of the Joint Commission on Mental Health to learn how people obtain psychiatric help in this country: most of it comes from persons outside the psychiatric profession. To take another example: the nursing profession has negotiated statutory licensing in every state of the union, but nevertheless there have evolved new categories of persons who perform nursing tasks. Licensing alone is no guarantee of control.

The fifth proposal urges job specifications for ancillary personnel, i.e., clear definition of the functions to be assigned the less trained. How practical is this in an open society? Will any administrator be bound by such arbitrary regulations? To maximize agency output with the budget at his disposal, he must utilize personnel as effectively and imaginatively as possible; he cannot suppress the exercise of intelligence or disregard experience gained on the job. Once the law is altered to reduce malpractice and negligence suits, the administrator will be even more inclined to give a heavier weight to experience than to training.

A realistic strategy in manpower planning is to act with respect to the more egregious problems. This is the substance of the next point of the report, which recommends an improvement in the salary scale and enhancement of career opportunities. It should be apparent, however, that the limiting factor is the assessment made by employers—voluntary agencies, boards, and legislators—of the unique contributions of different professions and skills. Today, the federal government pays $25,000 to senior scientists, but it pays considerably less to senior social workers. Right or wrong, this is Congress' estimate of the relative contributions of the two groups and, in an open society, such determinations must be made by the market or the legislature.

The final recommendation is aimed at manpower fact-finding. This appears to be less important and less useful than research into the effectiveness with which social workers perform. Studies of the latter type have thus far been largely neglected.

Perspective on solving manpower problems must await clarification and resolution of certain conflicts and contradictions that pervade the field of welfare. All of the helping professions, from psychiatry to those who attempt to provide assistance to the indigenous poor, are caught by a failure to clarify the source of the principal strengths of those who provide the service—is it their character, their education, or their experience that is the critical factor?

To pursue this matter a little further: Psychiatric nurses have had considerable specialized training, but in light of the rigidity of nursing education, is it the optimal training for work with mentally ill patients? A distinguished psychiatrist once remarked that the best mental hospital he had ever seen was an institution with 1,800 patients which had no psychiatrist on the staff. When asked what constituted the appropriate educational background of a good

ward attendant, another distinguished psychiatrist remarked, "Enough to make sure that he doesn't give the
patient the wrong medicine." That implies that a minimum level of literacy will suffice. Critically important are
personality characteristics. A ward attendant must like
people and not be afraid of illness.

We are pursuing a mirage in our indiscriminate emphasis on formal learning in the selection of all categories of
personnel. In the course of professionalization, social work
and the helping fields generally have underestimated the
relevance of empathy and experience. Recent graduates of
schools of social work who confront for the first time Southern rural Negroes or whites are much less able to make
effective contact with them than a sympathetic middle-aged
school teacher who has been working in the South.

All helping fields suffer from another difficulty—the inability to assess with any exactitude the relationship between input and output, whether their actions and programs have a positive, neutral, or negative effect. This
important, if unpleasant, fact is true of medicine, psychiatry, counseling, social work, psychology, the ministry. We
have few criteria and fewer techniques for evaluation, and
while this might presage a certain amount of modesty and
tentativeness, it also contributes to overreaction and excessive claims.

Social work has three distinguishable functions: to provide information and material resources to people in need;
to help people negotiate more effectively the complex institutions of our society; and to try to modify their behavior
patterns. These functions may not be of the same order of

importance. But training future workers depends on clarification.

A related question concerns the soundness of a generic
education, given the differences that exist between casework, medical social work, community work, group work,
social welfare administration, psychiatric social work, and
the various other subspecialties. To what extent does a core
program have relevance for areas that are so distinct?

The multiplicity of working relationships and organizational forms in social work practice is also a challenge to
training. Scanning the literature, one encounters many
models. Sometimes a social worker is seen as a member of
an institutional team where she mediates between the hospital and the family, between the patient and the staff.
Other models see the social worker as head of a large team
with various specialists assisting in the accomplishment of
her work. This is less familiar. And then a large part of
social work continues to involve the classic one-to-one
worker-client relationship. Unless these different methods
of work are much more sharply differentiated, education
and training will founder. To formulate an extreme position: graduate schools should stress the management of
social organizations that provide services for large numbers
of people. If this were accepted it would imply a curriculum built around such areas as budgeting, research, evaluation techniques, hiring and inservice training—in other
words, managerial skills. However, there is little evidence
that the profession is willing to move so radically.

Assuming the continuation of generic social work education, we confront an old area of conflict: what should

serve as the intellectual underpinning? Is psychology the core element in education for social work or are sociology, economics, and political science preferred fare?

Many issues have been identified and many leads have been opened up to clarify the uncertainties that surround them. In this concluding section an effort will be made to narrow the discussion to avoid unnecessary misunderstanding.

First, there are many closely related fields, each one of which finds its rationale in "helping people." Second, it is impossible to delineate a unique area for social work. Third, when necessary, employers will use anybody and everybody who can perform the work that is required and will show preference for those to whom they can pay the least. American society does not consider social work a distinctive and unique area. Our society wants more social workers, but it will never delegate to the profession the type of controls that it permits physicians to exercise.

Against this background, how should the profession move on the manpower front? If it sincerely wishes to provide more services for more people, and the Congress and the state legislatures concur, it must focus its attention not only on the college level, but also at the junior college and community college level. It should make a more strenuous effort to encourage the establishment of undergraduate training programs with a major in social work in as many public and private colleges as possible, with special attention to institutions in regions which now suffer from acute shortages of social work staff.

The challenge with respect to junior colleges consists of

defining more clearly the functions that a social work technician can effectively discharge, to develop appropriate curricula for the training of such technicians, and to work for their adoption in a large number of institutions.

At the master's and doctoral levels, the most serious problem appears to be a shortage of teaching and supervisory staff, for which there is no easy solution. One expedient might be to devise more combined programs with appropriate university departments, particularly government, sociology, and economics.

There is need for much more on-the-job training, with an aim at economies in supervision. Since the work that is performed differs from one agency to the next and from one program to the next within the same agency, considerable training must inevitably take place on the job. Most people who enter social work have a deep interest in the field and have the capacity to learn quickly in a concrete work situation. More advantage should be taken of this fact.

If social work is intervention aimed at helping large numbers of people in need, we cannot continue a system of graduate training oriented toward services to the individual. It is precious, inadequate, anachronistic. At a minimum, doctoral candidates should be educated as potential managers of large welfare organizations and as planners and research workers. There may be an insatiable demand for more casework, but this should not be the primary focus of graduate instruction.

There is obviously need for operational research. There is little systematic information about who applies for services, who gets them, and the results which accrue.

Social work has long realized that perhaps its unique quality is to relate for people in need one part of the complex social system to another. But it has not yet acted on this insight. It must seek to multiply its effectiveness by making alliances with other groups. To illustrate: in a democracy, when there is a long-term discrepancy between the resources available and the services required, it is the obligation of every profession to explore new ways of closing the gap. If they do not respond, if they withdraw behind the cloak of professionalism, some other group will move into the breach.

PART FOUR

Sickness and
Society

❧15❧
The Mentally Handicapped

In recent years we have begun to recognize that many persons suffering from handicaps and disabilities are as much the concern of the social scientist as the physician, for their ability to function may depend more on the environment than on medical diagnosis and therapy. The mentally handicapped comprise a large group whose condition is, more often than not, more social than medical.

When dealing with such complex phenomena as the mentally retarded persons, those who suffer from mental illness, delinquents, or any other large pathological constellation, it is often difficult to separate the genetic from the environmental components.

In our country we like to deal in large figures. We blow up our categories in order to get public attention and, we hope, public action. We talk about the tens of millions of people who have chronic illness. We talk about fifteen to twenty million people who are emotionally unstable. We talk about the many millions who are alcoholics. What do these figures mean? Although a great many people drink too much, it is impossible to count them. Similarly, to talk about five million mentally retarded persons is almost meaningless.

One can also question the logic of arbitrarily dividing people on a continuum of an intelligence scale into discrete categories. What do we know about the significant differences that are embedded in test scores of 65 and 50?

The outsider is also disturbed because five million human beings are all subsumed under the description of mental retardation, even though we understand the etiology of not more than 20 to 25 percent of the total group. We have defined a population but we lack diagnostic tools with which to distinguish among the members. The literature does not sharply delineate between severely retarded human beings, who need constant supervision and high orders of protection, and people who live in the community but who have difficulty in operating effectively in a competitive society.

Earlier studies by the Conservation of Human Resources Project at Columbia University and a more recent analysis of young men rejected for military service by the President's Task Force on Manpower Conservation (*One Third of the Nation*, 1964) provide interesting and insightful observations into the pathology of the mentally handicapped.[1] On the basis of our studies of *The Uneducated* and *The Ineffective Soldier*,[2] we can extract the following:

There was more than an eightfold variation among the nine regions of the country in the percentages of men who were rejected for military service because of mental deficiency during World War II.

The average rejection rate for Negroes was about six times that for whites.

But the regional variability among rejection rates for

both whites and Negroes was of the order of fivefold.
On a state basis the variability for whites was from a low
of 5 per 1,000 in Washington and Oregon to 55 per 1,000
in Kentucky, Tennessee, and North Carolina; the range
among Negroes was eightfold, from 36 in New York
State to 277 in South Carolina.

As the foregoing makes clear the rejection rate for
Negroes in New York was considerably below the white
rate for several Southern states.

The criterion used for rejection for mental or educational deficiency in World War II was the ability to read
and write at fifth-grade level. Men who did not meet this
criterion were classified as illiterate. In the intervening
years, the armed services were less pressed for manpower,
their equipment had become more technical, and their
tasks more complicated. Consequently they raised their
literacy requirements from the fifth-grade to eighth-grade
level.

On the basis of this criterion what do we find? *One-
Third of a Nation* reported that one-third of all youngsters
reaching 18 are rejected by the armed services for medical,
mental, or administrative reasons. Of those rejected for
mental or educational deficiency, about half are rejected
because they fail the Armed Forces Qualification Test
(AFQT). That is, one-half of one-third, or one-sixth, of
the draft-eligible 18-year-olds are rejected for military
service because they do not meet the criterion of the
equivalent of an eighth-grade level of schooling.

Once again the variability among the states is great.
There is a 20 to 1 difference. In some of the states, such as

South Carolina and Mississippi, 1 out of every 2 young men liable for military service is rejected because of a mental handicap. This figure applies to the total group of selectees, Negroes and whites combined. In Minnesota and in the states of the Northwest, under 3 percent are rejected. While the Negro rates have not been published separately in this report we learn from other data that about 3 out of 4 Negroes in the Deep South appearing for the examination cannot pass the eighth-grade test.

Although many of the facts we want to know remain obscure, there is one conclusion that is clear and unequivocal. An interpretation of mental deficiency based on race is not supported by these figures. While it is true that the average rate of white rejections is far below the Negro average, rates of rejection of Negroes in some northern states in World War II, and currently, are below the rates of rejection of the white population in some states in the South. Interestingly enough, that was true even in World War I.

In our study of *The Uneducated* we computed three factors for each state: educational expenditures, per capita income, and the degree of rurality. We found that there was a close relationship between these factors and rejection rates. The states with the lowest expenditures for education had seven times more rejections than those with the highest expenditures; the rich states had rejection rates equal to one-eighth that of the poor states; the rates for the urban areas were only one-seventh that of rural areas. These three basic factors, educational expenditures, per capita income, and rurality, explained most of the variability among the states.

One-Third of a Nation reported that 2 out of 5 of the youths rejected on the basis of the AFQT never went beyond elementary school. Since the test requires achievement roughly the equivalent of the eighth grade, this is hardly surprising. The second finding is that 4 out of 5 rejectees did not finish high school. The third finding is that of those rejectees who were out of school, 1 out of 3 was unemployed. Since most of the selectees were 21 or 22, an unemployment rate of 33 percent is very high.

Two more interesting findings show up. In the United States as a whole, only one-third of all families have more than four children. But 7 out of 10 youths rejected for military service came from large families. One out of 2 came from families with six children or more. Only 10 percent of all the families in the United States have six or more children, but they contributed 50 percent of the rejectees. This unusual finding is even more significant when considered in conjunction with another piece of evidence: 1 out of 2 of the young men came from families with an income of less than $4,000; 1 out of 5 came from a family with an income of less than $2,000.

It begins to appear that there is a heavy cycle of poverty: parents at the lower end of the socioeconomic scale produce many youngsters who, in turn, do poorly in school, drop out, and consequently perform poorly. The one difference between the present and the earlier data is that 70 percent of the recent rejectees are urban-reared. It would be helpful to know whether these families were first generation migrants into urban centers. Social research has produced relatively little information on the differentiation of problem populations of urban centers. In general migrants have a particularly difficult time; they come into the cities from Southern farms, or even from Northern farms, and are handicapped in adjusting to modern city living. To what extent our urban problems arise from the problems of migrants and to what extent these problems are independent of migration has not been determined.

A similar question may be posed concerning the regional differences discussed earlier. It is known that since the Civil War the North and South have experienced differential immigration of Europeans. Only a small number of European immigrants settled in the South. Nevertheless, the population in the South increased at a rate almost equal to that of the North and the West, which gained many millions through immigration. The increase in the Southern population was achieved through a fantastic increase in the birth rate in the South after the Civil War. The major crop of the South has long been babies. The relationship between its expanding population and its other problems has not been fully explored.

These data set the stage for a consideration of the employment of the mentally handicapped. The founder of economics, Adam Smith, begins his great book *The Wealth of Nations* with the statement that the skill and dexterity of the population is the key to the wealth of a nation. There is always a mutual accommodation between an economy and the qualities of the population. In 1945, Peking was a city of a million and a half or two million. If a U.S. military vehicle broke down in Peking at that time, the only persons able to fix it were Japanese prisoners of war. There are undoubtedly native-born mechanics in Peking today.

The interplay between demand for and availability of skill helps to explain why in World War I the U.S. Army rejected only about 40,000 men because of mental deficiency while for a force only three times as large in World War II almost 2 million were put in this category. The educational level of the population is constantly rising, but so are the skill needs of the economy and the military. However, the two must remain more or less in tandem. In the Korean War, for instance, the armed services found that much signal equipment was not used because it was overengineered and the soldiers preferred World War II equipment. Imbalances can occur, but the skill requirements of the economy tend to rise in consonance with the increasing competences of the population.

Our present society depends on many technical gadgets that produce difficulties for the mentally handicapped. Apartment houses are furnished with gas stoves. This presupposes that people know when to turn off the gas. In an agricultural society of an earlier day, the opportunities for simple-minded people, or just simple people, to get into trouble were much less. The fact that we murder over 50,000 people a year on the highways is an indication of an imbalance between technology and the emotional maturity, if not the intellectual maturity, of our population. A large number of the people who annually lose their lives on the highways are killed because we have more powerful instruments in the hands of the population than the population is competent to deal with.

Historically the farm was able to absorb people with

limited competence because it provided opportunities for the mastery of tasks requiring different amounts of skill and energy. For example, a person who is unbalanced emotionally or one who is not coordinated enough to remember to button his trousers creates no problem on a farm. But such a man cannot live in a city. The police will pick him up. An urban civilization makes demands on conformity. The farm is a preferred environment to absorb people with limited competence.

In our study of *The Ineffective Soldier* there are several life histories that indicate how protective a farm environment is for simple people. Several young men reported that they went to a movie once or twice a year and lived close to their parents the rest of the time. That is not possible in a city. Many farm youths with limited competence have moved into Chicago and New York with resulting problems of adjustment and control.

One reason for the migration to the cities is automation, a scare term for technological change. Successive technological changes have eliminated many of the simple jobs on the farm and have reduced drastically the amount of unskilled labor required. The equipment is expensive and simple-minded persons cannot operate it. Automation has also permeated manufacturing and eliminated not only unskilled jobs but also many semiskilled jobs. We are beginning to use more and more machines in white-collar and office work. A large number of jobs of routine, repetitive nature are being eliminated. Fortunately for the mentally handicapped, machines cannot be used throughout all the service sector of the economy. On the other hand, it is difficult to supervise and control employees in the service sector, and this explains why so much service is of poor quality.

An affluent society, with its high income levels, heavy use of capital equipment, and sophisticated demand for quality output finds it increasingly difficult to absorb unskilled labor. The fact that we work increasingly in large organizations creates additional demands: an employee must learn how to adjust to a large number of different supervisors and fellow workers. Many of the soldiers who broke down in the armed services found the complex military society more than they could cope with.

Another factor that will have an adverse effect on individuals with low mental achievement is the job situation. Despite our continuing prosperity, the employment situation is unfavorable for these people. Ours is an economy that has less and less need to hire young people. Employers realize that young people are likely to be unstable since they are searching for congenial work and favorable conditions of employment. Unless they have to, employers try to avoid hiring young people. This helps to explain our persistently high rates of unemployment among teenagers.

In a loose labor market the employer is in a preferred position to pick and choose. Large employers with preferred jobs have long had selective hiring practices in their desire to protect their expensive capital equipment and their delicately articulated organization. The demand for people who have some difficulty in learning and some difficulty in performing is definitely limited.

A few points about research and action. The United

States is now committed to a new dimension of social policy, which goes under the loose heading of a "war on poverty." We are trying to mitigate conditions for those at the lower end of the income distribution. It does not matter whether there are twenty-five million or thirty million involved here, there are too many people with too little income.

We need to learn more about how to help the poor and to enable them to help themselves. We need to learn more about the antecedent factors involved in poverty and the consequences poverty brings with it. We need epidemiological studies that will throw new light on the mentally handicapped. In connection with the new programs being launched in Appalachia, we should seek to learn about the distribution of capacities of youngsters of different ages growing up under seriously adverse circumstances.

It is important to isolate the effects of genetic components, family relationships, and community characteristics on the ultimate functioning of the individual. It is not easy to differentiate among the community and the family and the individual's inheritance, but we should try to. One of the serious problems of the mentally handicapped is that often they have multiple disabilities. We learned in World War II that an individual with one handicap could make a reasonable adjustment in the Army. But it was difficult to find a place in the system for men with multiple handicaps. This suggests a research clue: it may be that many who show up later in life as mentally handicapped (educationally deprived) are actually reflecting an antecedent handicap that was not picked up. This includes youngsters who cannot hear or see properly in the classroom as well as those who are too disturbed to adjust. These antecedent factors may make learning difficult if not impossible. Ordering of multiple handicaps suggests the importance of early diagnosis and establishing priorities for intervention.

Our increasing national affluence should lead us to commit more of our wealth to those who need help. It is indecent for a society of two-car families to look forward to becoming a society of three-car families. At some stage the acquisition of additional appurtenances of wealth is not a desideratum. We may choke to death from the fumes of our many machines. While we still have the opportunity we should consider the services that many people need, and their priority. A civilized society must be concerned with the people within it who start life with severe handicaps and who require special assistance.

The outlook for the employment of the mentally handicapped is not propitious. The literature dealing with the vocational rehabilitation of the mentally retarded is not encouraging. But the outlook can be changed. If we have a large pool of handicapped persons and start a new vocational rehabilitation program, we skim the top and almost always get good returns. In a complex economy with 80 million jobs, we can make room for a few thousand handicapped people and show good results. A critical question is the degree of effort, energy, and cooperation that is needed to feed these few in. To integrate large numbers of severely handicapped into a competitive economy does not appear feasible.

The best way to get social action in a democracy is to

organize the largest possible group of claimants. We have a society with many who are emotionally unbalanced to a point where they cannot be integrated into a large organization. Some may have an IQ of 160 but they do not fit in. There are large numbers with severe physical handicaps. We have large numbers of older people, and will have more of them, who have less physical strength and poorer educational qualifications than the younger group coming into the labor market. The total constituency of handicapped people is sizable.

If we disregard for the moment the nature of the person's handicap and simply argue that everybody is entitled to a chance to make a contribution to the society of which he is a part, then we can state that a rich society has an obligation to create reasonable opportunities for all who desire and are able to participate constructively. It may not be feasible to do this in terms of a competitive market place. But it should be feasible to do it within a noncompetitive structure. This is a major challenge to government. We need a political commitment to this goal and we need the intellectual imagination to structure a protected market, where large numbers of people with handicaps can work at 70 percent of capacity, 60 percent of capacity, even 40 percent in useful jobs, jobs that society wants done and where the costs of supervision are not excessive. There will come a point where the costs of managing the severely handicapped may be disproportionate, but we are far from that.

It would be foolish to claim that it will be easy to organize the many types of protected environments that would be required if we were to make a serious effort to open employment opportunities for all of the handicapped, or even for most of them. We noted earlier that the educational and skill requirements in our society continue to increase. And yet there are different ways of performing work. If our objective were to maximize the number of jobs available for the hard-to-employ we might go about the problems of industrial engineering and organizational management quite differently from the manner in which an employer bent on maximizing his profits approaches his task. The more the pursuit of profits results in a larger surplus, the more we should feel under obligation to redirect part of that surplus to provide a more meaningful life for those whom fate has short-changed.

We have to develop more institutions which will be able to employ people under less than fully competitive circumstances. First, we must conceive of their problems as not exclusively medical or biological or genetic, and surely not primarily or solely economic or social. The problem of fitting them in is one to which all of the disciplines can contribute. Economics is in a particularly good position since it is above all else concerned with work—with inputs of effort and with social benefits. While we are looking for more knowledge of the causes of deficiency, we can do much to ameliorate the problems of the mentally handicapped by providing them the opportunity to work at the level of their competence.

❧ 16 ❧

Priorities for Psychiatry

It was World War II that put psychiatry on the map in the United States. Thousands of physicians, most of them with no more than a 90-day conversion course, were given the task of helping millions of soldiers tolerate the stresses and strains of military, particularly combat, conditions. A new world of the psyche was revealed to these former internists, surgeons, obstetricians, pediatricians—as well as to the old-fashioned psychiatrists who, up to that point, had equated their discipline with keeping seriously disturbed persons under lock and key in out-of-the-way hospitals. They too began, as a result of their military experience, to dream of a new world where psychiatry could be as therapeutic as the other medical specialties.

As is so frequently the case with revolutions, enthusiasm carried everything before it until the leaders of the profession convinced not only themselves but the American people as well, that a new day had dawned and that with proper financing and support, psychiatry would "pay off." But most of the leaders had little interest in or understanding of the political and economic realities to which legislators had to remain responsive. And so, after a time, disillusionment began to set in.

In this chapter an effort will be made to carry through a point-counterpoint analysis of the political realities as they bump against professional practices out of which we will, we hope, gain a sharper insight into priorities for psychiatry in a real rather than ideal world.

Politics versus Psychiatry

1. Whenever a service preempts as large a proportion of a state budget as does education or mental health, it can be anticipated that not much change will occur from year to year. This is an elementary rule of budgeting logistics and an important one to remember for planning and policy determination.

2. Psychiatric care, like medical care generally, is a service, not a commodity. The significance of this distinction lies in the fact that the delivery of services is mediated exclusively by people—practitioners, whose availability will largely determine the success or failure of any program. In a free society there are many different streams of money which provide multiple options to individuals; thus, simply to increase any one stream will not insure that competent personnel will be available at the proper place to perform specific services for which the funds have been designated. This is our initial experience with Medicare and Medicaid. Federal funds for health have been substantially increased with no commensurate increase in the provision of health services to people who did not have them previously. In an open market, consumers with more money always compete

with those who have less; given a limited supply of resources, the scarcer services will tend to go to the affluent.
This is true even in socialist countries; patients who can
pay or who are powerful get better attention.

3. A wave of optimism has accompanied the concept of
community mental health centers, community-based treatment services, and the literature reflects considerable pressure for the imminent replacement of the existing mental
hospital system with these new types of facilities. A cautionary note should be struck. The legislatures of the several
states have invested large sums in physical plants which,
from an economist's point of view, represent sunk costs,
subject to modification only over time as new funds become
available. Alternatively, as extensions or additions to plants
are built, they may incorporate new principles and new
ideas. The expectation, however, that our large mental hospitals will be abandoned and that we shall develop a radically different physical structure is simply not realistic. The
constraints imposed by capital investment are no less relevant for state legislatures than they are for private business.
Major institutional changes, such as plant relocation or
basic functional alterations, can occur only gradually, in
response to obsolescence, population shifts, and other long-
term forces.

4. An intrinsic characteristic of all services is the difficulty of measuring performance, a problem that particularly confounds education. Legislators who appropriate
money, and particularly the citizens to whom they must
answer, are keenly aware of the broad scope that exists for

deciding whether a program or institution is good, adequate, passable, or inferior.

There is an amazing range in the costs and charges of different types of mental institutions. A well-run private hospital may charge from $15,000 to $25,000 a year for custodial care and little more. At the opposite extreme are some good state mental hospitals with a broad spectrum of therapeutic treatment for newly admitted patients for whom the average cost is about $3,000 annually.

As long as expenditures are at a level which protects patients from gross neglect and abuse, it is difficult to justify additional expenditures to the public unless they can be related to quantifiable gains, such as shorter hospitalization and more recoveries.

And an honest administrator will admit that if the legislature had allowed him not $2,000 but $4,000 per patient per year, he could not guarantee that his performance record would be significantly improved. Mental illness is too elusive to yield directly to additional financial, even therapeutic inputs.

5. In certain fields, particularly in social programing, supply tends to create its own demand. Even a substantial increase in the number of people who provide a service may not close the gap. The critical question is what happens in the interim to expectations? If they increase faster than the resources the gap will in fact widen. As conditions in financing health care change, people who formerly suffered medical neglect begin actively to seek care. Much the same dynamic can be found in connection with poverty.

Since standards change it is simplistic to believe that an open society can ever eliminate deprivation, because it is always relative. The relativity of criteria of need is dramatically evident in the case of, for example, Ethiopia, a country where the average per capita income is under $50 per year. On this incredibly small sum, most Ethiopians manage to live, eat, and have some fun. Here in the United States with $4,000 annually, we should be vastly better off. But are we? Since rising incomes bring rising expectations, the demand for additional health and welfare services may increase rather than decline and we shall continue to experience many shortages.

6. The definition of health adopted by the World Health Organization, which includes not only freedom from disease but optimal functioning for all people, is useful only as an ideal. The gap between reality and the ideal is great, even in rich nations, and under this definition it will inevitably remain large, since optimal functioning involves subjective as well as objective criteria of well-being. Therefore this definition is not operationally useful when it is applied to nations which are lower on the wealth and income distribution scale. The definition further blurs the position of health since optimal functioning involves as well all the other dimensions of human life—economic, social, political, educational, cultural.

7. This open-ended character of demand for medical services reinforces the skepticism of a legislature when approached for additional funds. If the lawmakers believe that patients are receiving reasonable care they are disinclined to vote additional funds unless the public demands

them. State services can always be improved, but only if the taxpayers will tolerate additional taxes.

8. The various health professions seem overinvolved in competitive struggles when they might be more productively occupied in complementing each other's activities with an aim of ameliorating gross shortages. The proceedings of a conference in a Northeastern state on psychiatric social work and public health nursing have recently been published. It is a discouraging record. Public health nurses and psychiatric social workers debated functional boundaries over which neither group had any real control. The debate reflects the fact that ours is an open society which allows freedom to groups to stake out their respective claims. In contrast, the military does not face this problem. Rank and authority decide questions of function and boundaries, the assignment system is controlled, and an effort is made—although it frequently does not succeed—to utilize people so that their skills will complement each other. But in civilian life we have an open system built on competition which is usually directed at raising educational requirements without much consideration of their relevance for performance. At the present time, salaries and functional assignments in most professional fields are determined on the basis of educational achievement with the result that many individuals are arbitrarily prohibited from doing work for which they are often well qualified.

The market, however, exercises a degree of corrective influence. The nursing field, which has suffered a chronic shortage since World War II, illustrates this well. While the leaders of the profession have concentrated upon raising educational requirements, actual pressures have produced a large increase in the number of practical nurses with less qualifications than registered nurses. The compulsive influence of the market has affected psychiatry in much the same way. Though the profession has been highly exclusionary, literally tens of thousands of untrained, partially trained, and nonmedically trained psychotherapists have entered the field and are now in active, profitable and, it is hoped, useful practice.

9. Our system of federal funding for medical care is far from satisfactory, particularly from the point of view of the states. While the concept of categorical grants may be justified at the initiation of a program, these should not be continued indefinitely. It is not wise for the federal government to seek to determine local programs. Offering money to the states specifically for programs that have the approval of Washington does not necessarily add strength to our national system. It would be preferable to require the states to draw up a one-, three-, or five-year plan dictated by local needs and to submit such a plan for federal review against established criteria. Once these have been satisfied, funds should be released to the state authorities, who would then have the responsibility for providing various services.

10. Several friends of psychiatry warned some years ago against the dangers of overselling it. All struggles for budget are competitive: mental health, welfare, education. Each campaigns for a larger stake, which each attempts to justify with extravagant claims. Would it not be more judicious at this time to evaluate thoroughly the aims, the goals, the mission of psychiatry? To distinguish clearly the core

from the periphery? Unless claims are restricted to the essential, the unambiguous, and the justifiable, attempts to obtain additional resources will probably be frustrated.

In this connection it is important to note that the public is ambivalent toward mental disease and psychiatry. A large part of our population knows that a person who becomes mentally ill may or may not recover, that there are serious mental illnesses which are not subject to cure, some not even to alleviation. The public also knows that, psychoses aside, many people manage to cope with their emotional problems. Though they need help, it is not always clear who can help them and whether the cost will be justified for the modest help they can anticipate. These considerations suggest the importance of modest claims by the mental health movement.

Problem Areas

Against the background of these general observations, we can look at selected problems in the field of mental health. To begin with the question of claims: many articulate psychiatrists have repeatedly testified before Congress about significant therapeutic advances. But we must question whether there is solid evidence, reinforced by follow-up, to support such claims. Admittedly, state hospital census figures are down, not up; yet there has been an upward drift in patient admissions figures. But the total system has been changing and we now treat many patients in new kinds of settings. Are they included in the totals? Another reason for caution is the readmission rate. Still another is what happens to the patient who is discharged. Is his recovery maintained? Not much is known. To release a patient from the hospital is easier than to absorb him at home. And without adequate follow-up data, we remain in the dark. Consider, for instance, a mother whose depression is not really over when she is released (on improved status) to her home to care for her children. How can we be sure that the drop in hospital census resulted, in fact, in a net social gain?

The concept of community mental health centers has been widely and enthusiastically received, more on grounds —thus far—of theory than of experience. Ultimately, these programs may justify all the claims made for them in the areas of primary and secondary prevention. At present, however, the danger exists that distinctions between mild and more profound disorders may become blurred in the initial experimentation with new agencies and new programs. It would be a mistake if the limited attention now directed to the psychoses, which remain the most critical unresolved problem in psychiatry, were further reduced.

How do these several matters relate to manpower problems and their possible solutions? Insufficient attention has been given to the potentialities of alternative staffing patterns. What are the advantages of struggling to add a few more psychiatrists to a hospital staff over utilizing the funds for salaries to train and upgrade attendants? On balance, it might prove more productive to upgrade the attendants. It would surely be more effective to institute a career system for attendants. Otherwise, the currently high turnover

rates will persist, and poor hospital care will be perpetu-
ated, irrespective of the number of psychiatrists.

This imbalance in staffing is not unique to mental institutions. We see it in general hospitals as well, which often
have a full complement of physicians but insufficient nurses
and aides to provide good patient care. One reason that we
encounter so little imaginative planning, so few original
approaches to the ubiquitous staffing problems, is that the
individual who eventually heads a large hospital (and this
is particularly true of psychiatric hospitals) is more often
than not a physician who has received little training in
administration and the management of ancillary personnel
in the course of his medical training. Therefore he is likely
to follow the staffing patterns he inherited, making ad hoc
changes only. This is scarcely an effective strategy for organizational survival and improvement.

It does not follow that the person who has had the best
training in a discipline is necessarily the best person to care
for a patient. In light of the former emphasis on depth psychology and the new emphasis on chemotherapy in the
teaching of psychiatrists, it may well be the psychiatric social worker who has the most to offer certain types of patients, especially those with reality problems. In this connection, it should be noted that choice of therapy depends
on manpower. Most cardiac patients must be treated without recourse to open heart surgery. At any given time the
preferred therapy is in part a function of the manpower
resources available.

If the trend continues for psychiatry to define as within
its province every individual who confronts emotional diffi-

culties, it will be necessary for the profession to liberalize its concept of staff. Clearly there will never be a sufficient number of trained psychiatrists to provide services for all who are emotionally disturbed. Only by involving teachers, ministers, judges, and other professionals can psychiatry conceivably meet such a broad commitment.

One of the dangers in mental health, as in other dynamic fields, is the temptation to neglect the older, more resistant problems in favor of currently exciting ones. Fashions influence medicine and science no less than they influence other fields. We have seen public health undergo several distinct shifts in interest—from infectious disease control to radiation problems and now air pollution. A specialty such as mental health, which deals essentially with chronic illness, may find the attraction of the new more compelling than the old. How to work with a group of mentally retarded youngsters so that they can be helped to adjust within the community at a minimal level may not be exciting, but it may be very important.

Policy Alternatives

Now a few comments relevant to policy. It is probably no longer valid to think in terms of the mental hospital population as a totality; instead discussion and planning should focus on specific categories of patients. There are the senile, the arteriosclerotic, and other individuals with organic impairment which is irreversible. There are alcoholics and the narcotic patients for whom we have no effective psychotherapy, and who are often regarded as social rather than psychiatric problems. The key challenge remains the young and the middle-aged psychotic patient. How many can be helped with proper treatment to recover and be restored to normal function? How many of these will relapse and be added to the slowly accumulating chronic population? It is an error to consider an undifferentiated mental hospital patient load because of the wide differences in prognosis, needs, and goals.

Improved social security benefits, Medicare and Medicaid, and chemotherapy may act to slow the increasing hospitalization of the aged in mental institutions. And of those requiring intramural care, at least part of the inflow is likely to be absorbed by nursing homes.

Despite the large research funds that have been available to the National Institute of Mental Health, we know much less than we should about the discharged mental patient. The importance of systematic follow-up is essential if we are to learn what happens during the course of a total illness within a hospital and outside.

Further challenge and opportunity exist to help people outside exclusively psychiatric confines, specifically in improved liaison between mental health and interested governmental departments, such as welfare, public health, education, and labor. Current concepts of treatment of mental illness place increasing stress on social criteria of recovery. No patient can be cured or his problem solved in isolation. Instead all the instruments of society should be mobilized to help restore him to effective social functioning, and chief among these are education, training, and employment. It seems clear that a patient's recovery can never be completed either by the physician or the mental hospital or the two in combination. At best their function is preparatory to a broader social resolution.

Given such a comprehensive mandate, the state departments of mental health should be granted as much administrative freedom as possible so that they can utilize their funds and their manpower more effectively. The difficulties of operating in a manpower-short economy are compounded by regulations that restrict utilizing the manpower that is available.

In brief recapitulation, the significant questions leaders of the mental health movement today must face are: What do they *really* know about the effectiveness of current efforts? What do they *really* need to find out in order to assess their programs? What can they *really* hope to do? What do they *really* need by way of resources?

The field faces a great many manpower problems. But before seeking additional manpower, it is essential that the leadership define more sharply its primary and secondary missions, and to determine what is feasible and what is not. The public purse is limited; the nation's manpower resources must be allocated among a great many competing purposes. Psychiatry is entitled to its share, but neither psychiatry nor any other field can hope to obtain more resources than will meet its priority needs.

❧17❧

Mental Health in Industry

American industry, its structure, its technology, and its conditions of employment, are repeatedly cited as a growing, barely restrainable pathogen threatening the mental health of its vast number of employees. How true is this?

In the attempt to formulate an approach to the question of mental health within our industrial structure, a series of tension points emerging from the changing structure of work have been identified. At the same time, the possibilities of adjustment that exist within an employment arena are explored.

The ten possible sources of tension described here do not represent a major drift toward generalized pathology. Nevertheless, they represent potential increases in tension that are likely to be derivatives of current alterations in the work scene.

Although we need not be unduly concerned about the effects of technological changes and automation on the nature of manufacturing and on some of the service sectors, the work place may in the future be a less sociable environment. There will probably be less direct association between worker and worker and between worker and supervisor. There will be more space, more distance, and more isolation, and this may create tension for people who do not like isolation.

The reverse is also true: those who like to be alone will find the work environment more satisfactory. In one study of industrial psychology a worker achieved "mental equilibrium" only after he became a night driver for a milk company. This was his ideal adjustment. Each change affects each worker differently. But on the assumption that most people find in work support from close association with others and that Americans in particular find isolation and quiet difficult, there may be more tension in the work place in the future arising from increased isolation.

As more funds are invested in capital equipment, in complicated machines where the possibility of damage is tremendous, the quality of supervision, even indirect supervision, will be tightened. That may be burdensome to some workers. But other workers will enjoy the greater responsibility which may be associated with an improved work adjustment.

It is clear from recent prospective developments that there will be more Negroes and members of other minority groups hired, even as supervisors, in work places where traditionally they have not been employed as equals. This may create some tension for some who are deeply prejudiced. There will probably be more women, and more women in supervisory positions, which may create some tension for men and/or other women.

We will probably see an end to the current pattern of companies' hiring young people and saying to them, "Work hard for us and we will take care of you until you are ready to retire." This pattern of career insurance is not likely to be continued indefinitely in the future. The nature of management's problems in a rapidly changing technological and economic environment implies that management will have less and less interest in retaining a large number of older people, and the bonds between management and a large part of the work force will loosen. There was evidence of this in the steel industry a few years ago; also when Westinghouse found its profits declining; and in the petroleum industry which ran into difficulty in the late 1950s. In each instance, many people were let out early, including people high in management.

A large proportion of the men in gray flannel suits and their female counterparts—men and women who work in the higher echelons of large enterprises—have accumulated capital through organizational linkages and connections rather than in terms of market skills and competences. This is quite different from the old days, when a craftsman had his security in his toolbox. Today a man acquires security by being in an organization for a number of years; he knows how it works and he knows with whom to work. But this makes him somewhat vulnerable if he is displaced. A man may be worth $20,000 to a particular organization, but if he loses that job, he may not be worth $2,000 to another.

As organizations become national or international, it is more likely that people will feel lost. A considerable number of young executives leave large organizations, even though they have good futures in front of them, because they do not like to be anonymous.

Many marriages cannot withstand the necessity often incumbent upon young men to travel. For example, management consulting firms find it difficult to attract and hold staff because of the amount of traveling they require. At crucial times in the life cycle of a man, the necessity to travel, sometimes to relocate, can be disturbing.

The next point is somewhat in contradiction to the earlier one that people in large organizations acquire organizational capital. Attention is directed here to technically or scientifically trained people, of whom industry is hiring more and more. For these people, today's trend makes for new conflicts of values. By and large, the corporate structure looks for loyalty from its employees, but the better trained and educated people have a double affiliation, one to their discipline and one to their employer. This often creates tension for these individuals expressed by conflicts over publications of research policies.

As a function of our new affluence, we are, for the first time in the history of the world, close to the point where work, even for people who are seriously interested in their jobs, will absorb only a modest portion of our total energies. The work week is declining slowly but steadily. Before long we may be working a 32-hour week. Even today, some people—for example, airplane pilots—work only about 80 hours a month. The whole question of the pattern of life one wants to lead, and the balance between work and nonwork, is an interesting one. Possibly half of the American working population is already considerably more involved in the nonwork area of life than in their work. This does not mean that they are uninterested in their work, but that the importance of the work area is receding.

In a rapidly changing world in which knowledge and technology are making rapid gains, the premiums go to people who have been most recently trained. While there is always room for people with experience, a higher value is placed on the recent graduate, which is an inversion of the conventional pattern.

We are moving increasingly from a blue-collar to a white-collar economy. And in this move, there are implications for change in the pattern of slow promotions characteristic of the white-collar sector. Governmental employers now agree that their white-collar employees may unionize, although they are not supposed to strike. This reflects the fact that more and more white-collar workers believe they can bargain better collectively than individually. We can expect to see more trade-union activity in the white-collar area.

Even apart from the matter of trade unions the promotion possibilities for white-collar workers, who include high-school graduates, junior college graduates, college graduates, up to Ph.D. degree holders, will be increasingly limited unless these workers are offered a chance for further study and growth. A man who has a Ph.D. degree but no opportunity to continue to study because all of his time is preempted by his employer will be so far behind in his discipline within five or ten years that he might as well never have had completed his Ph.D. work. Keeping a white-collar force alive, interested, and concerned with its work will involve the employer in large investments in training time and effort.

At the turn of the century, when hordes of immigrants, foreigners, "greenhorns," illiterates, arrived on our shores, it was easy for an employer to take a high-handed view about his rights and the nonrights of his workers. At that time, an employer in Pennsylvania thought it would be a good idea to discharge his entire factory force one day and to rehire most but not all of them the next day, just to indicate who was boss.

In dealing with a more educated public—and the whole population is getting to be better educated—the question of arbitrariness takes on a different light. Consider the armed services today, which has a civilian board of military justice; or the insistence that the police no longer be a law unto themselves but have "civilian review boards." These are all facets of a much larger phenomenon in American life: to reduce, restrict, and constrain the arbitrariness of power. And as our work force becomes more educated, more sensitized, more developed, the more it will insist on restraining the power of the employer.

One of the ways to reduce tension points is to move toward objective systems of due process of law in disciplinary matters and areas of conflict between the individual and the organization. Even universities have been forced to realize that, if they want peace on the campus, provision must be made for machinery not only to adjudicate differences between the faculty and the administration but also to assign to the student body an appropriate role in all decision-making which relates to them.

People want, and have a right, in their own view and in the view of others, to be treated equitably. The drive toward equity cannot be minimized in a democratic society, and the potentialities for equitable treatment must be built into the system through more explicit personnel policies and more explicit criteria of evaluation.

One of the great strengths of large organizations is that they can provide more options for their workers. Options can reduce friction. During World War II, many servicemen studied Japanese and others studied French, but some who had studied French were shipped to Japan and others who had studied Japanese were shipped to France. A similar pattern exists in many large corporations. Large organizations are able to offer people options, but they are often reluctant to do so. Yet they would have many more satisfied employees if their workers had a role to play in decisions affecting them. A corporation cannot be run like a Greek democracy, but there is a middle ground between complete freedom of choice and no freedom of choice.

One area which could be improved is the training of the supervisory work force, particularly to alert them to the changing qualities of the workers. In the Army today, some sergeants still have an image of soldiers of twenty years ago —men who had finished eight grades of school or less. When they are confronted with men who have had two years of college, many cannot adjust.

The same situation prevails in many universities. There has been a sizable improvement in high-school teaching and in college teaching, but our graduate faculties have not adjusted adequately to the better quality of students.

The problem of enabling older supervisors to stay at-
tuned and sensitive to the changing quality of the people
they supervise is a complicated one. It is the same problem
that parents confront when they forget that children mature and continue to treat adolescents as if they were still
young children.

One of the unfortunate aspects of a large organization
is its need for generalized policy. But the need can be exaggerated. Management tends to preempt the discretionary
and judgmental factor that supervisors need to be effective.
If a supervisor has no scope for action, he is, in John Gard-
ner's apt phrase, "part of a Van Allen belt, through which
nothing can pass in either direction." Supervisors need
scope for discretion. They can then make distinctions among
people under their supervision, which they cannot do if
every step must be taken according to company-wide procedures.

The variety of work assignments in large corporations
offers one way of balancing the needs of people. Some jobs
require that people work closely with others. Other jobs
are quite isolated. There are jobs at night, jobs in the day-
time, jobs in small towns, jobs in big towns, jobs overseas,
etc. The full use of existing assignments in terms of the
satisfactions that they could yield or the dissatisfactions
they could create has not been understood.

Here, again, a military example may be useful. At certain stages in a man's life, it is easier for him to serve overseas than at others. If he has adolescent children who will
be in college in two years, it is a bad time to uproot him
and send him with his family overseas. If his youngsters are

already in college, he might be pleased, in fact he might prefer to move. Similar planning in business would require that corporations dovetail their needs with their employees' needs. But this can be done only if the company thinks it is important.

The support of management at times of personal crisis is a step toward humanity. We have learned that most people who break down psychologically recover. Many of them recover quickly and many might never break down if they receive a little support when they first confront a crisis. This reinforces the earlier plea for more discretion for supervisory personnel. Support for people at a strategic point and a little tolerance may cut substantially the costs of psychological breakdown or may even abort it.

Firmness of policy on issues where there may be conflict is important. For example, an important point for industry in the race issue is to avoid equivocation at the top. People down the line easily ferret out whether an executive means what he says or if he is merely talking. This is true even in a command organization such as the Army or the Catholic Church. Where there are known difficulties of securing agreement to new positions, top leadership has to make the investment of following through to obtain acquiescence and cooperation. The President of the United States can make a contribution to the nation's mental health by remaining in such a strong position with respect to the race issue that even the Deep South will finally understand that the country is committed to a policy of equality.

We still are in the early stages of a backwash of an unbounded enthusiasm for psychiatry. The Freudian revolution was one of the most important developments of the twentieth century. Dynamic psychology represents one of the important dimensions of contemporary thought. Nevertheless, over the last thirty years, more in some countries than in others and certainly in many parts of the United States, we have been on a psychological binge. My colleagues and I developed our critical position some years ago in a little volume called *The Optimistic Tradition and American Youth*.[1] We must not confuse everything bad in this world with mental illness and everything good with mental health. We need to keep some discriminations and some semantic differences. We need to know the differences among management's responsibilities, the physicians' responsibilities, and the individual's responsibilities.

Psychiatry is a branch of medicine. It is a specialty and its primary concern is the treatment and cure of mental illnesses. Regrettably, psychiatry is not able to treat or cure the scourge of psychosis because psychoses do not readily bend to treatment.

With regard to the neuroses, behavior defects and other personality disorders we are on quicksand. Admittedly many people are helped by some type of psychotherapy or chemotherapeutic treatment, but the arena remains undelineated and the criteria of evaluation are uncertain. Therefore circumspection is called for, particularly on the part of an employer.

When an individual decides to take some of his money and some of his time and seek psychiatric treatment it is a personal matter. The role of the organization is quite different. By and large, it is difficult to see a special role for psychiatry in industry other than as part of a medical department where it should operate as does any other medical specialty.

At one time it was thought that every large organization would have a place for a part-time, if not a full-time, psychiatrist, as an adviser to management for personnel and related matters. There are many reasons to question such an approach. It muddies the responsibility between line and staff. Supervisors should be responsible for making personnel judgments—whom to hire, promote, fire. Moreover, the question of confidentiality is relevant. If an employee consults the company psychiatrist and if the psychiatrist sees himself as a corporate official, he must decide what to pass on, what to hold in confidence.

The head of a monastery in Mexico reported at the Ecumenical Council that many members of his monastery had entered psychoanalytic treatment. He even had a woman as one of two analysts available to the brothers. The second report that he gave to the Council was that two-thirds of the members had resigned!

Some years ago the then chairman of the board of the Consolidated Edison Company of New York, Cyril Searing, was asked whether he had a psychiatrist on his staff. Mr. Searing answered, "Hell, no. The Board of Directors pays me $150,000 a year to run the organization and my job is to make sure that a lot of crazy people cooperate so that the organization runs. That's what they're paying me for." This comment indicates that the challenge for management is to coordinate the talents of many strong-willed people, each pulling in his own direction. There is no special role for the psychiatrist until somebody gives signs of becoming ill.

It is dangerous to bring into the work place criteria and assessments from the physician's office. The physician is able to make estimates about personality strengths and weaknesses because of a special therapeutic relationship. Dr. Else Brunswik once observed that the errors made by psychoanalysts and psychiatrists in military screening derived from the fact that they knew too much about the people they were assessing. It is possible to know too much as well as too little. Obviously, the performance of human beings is determined by more than their emotional constellation. It is determined also by organizational and environmental constraints and supports. The important point is that many neurotic people do a great deal of good work. It is dangerous to use psychiatric diagnostic categories for the assessment of potential performance. It could also be argued that the use of projective tests, psychiatric assessment, and psychological evaluations for employment and promotion are an invasion of privacy, a waste of the employer's money, and an intellectual fraud.

Since large sums of money are devoted to medical benefits for workers, management and trade unions might insist that these benefit programs include psychiatric treatment just as they include other medical treatment. Coverage for short-term psychiatric treatment has become increasingly common in Blue Cross programs. And looking ahead, we can expect to have more community psychiatry, more ambulatory treatment.

We cannot expect psychiatry to reduce labor–management conflicts. Even with an efficient management and an efficient trade union, there is room for conflict. The parties have real differences in goals, in values, and in objectives, and this is not the place for the psychiatrist to intervene.

There may be an occasional psychotic or borderline psychotic person in a position of power who can damage an organization but, in general, he reveals himself quickly and it is then up to the leadership to remove him. Unquestionably unstable bosses have destroyed people under them. But the removal of incompetent supervisors is a major task of top leadership.

Action Proposals

Role for psychiatry. There is a place for psychiatric services in industry just as there is a place for medical services in industry. There is a place for psychiatric services in medical programs that are paid for by trade unions and industry, jointly or individually.

Supervisory training. Some general psychological education for management might be helpful, such as teaching a group of first-line supervisors that human beings undergo periods of stress when they are more tense than at other times. But most people know this; it is whether they act on it that can spell the difference between a good supervisor and a poor one. Some formal training of supervisors may be desirable.

Need for factual data. Operational data about mental health in industry should be collected. How can pathology in organizations be identified; what are its manifestations?

How much malperformance is associated with mental illness?

Research on instability and work performance. Studies in depth might help us learn more about unstable people and their performance. Cooperative studies involving several organizations might also be undertaken. American industry, which has so much to its credit, undertakes too few cooperative studies, which would be of obvious advantage to all industry and the rest of the society, without any competitive disadvantage.

Economics of therapy and rehabilitation. Since much money is put into medical programs of one sort or another, it would be desirable to know about the cost of therapy and the cost of rehabilitation.

Absorbing hard-to-employ persons. In this country, we are at the beginning of a redefinition of our commitment to assure that every human being in our society who is capable of working has a chance to work. We will not continue to tolerate 5 percent unemployment and a much higher percentage of under-employment. We need more experimental programs particularly directed toward encouraging large employers in the private, nonprofit, and governmental sectors to modify the working environment to absorb more of the hard-to-employ. This group includes the mentally retarded, the emotionally unstable, the unskilled. We know too little about this large group with diversified handicaps.

If work is the major affirmative relationship of a human being to his society then we must do much more to provide jobs for all who want to work.

∾18∾

Tuberculosis Control

There are several points that inform an interested but not medically trained observer about tuberculosis. It is a disease which, despite substantial declines in both its morbidity and mortality rates, still abounds. While a spectacular breakthrough was made in therapy in the early 1950s which has been reflected in a marked drop in hospital bed requirements in the United States and in many other countries, it has been difficult to the point of exasperation to bring the full force of the new therapeutics into play.

In no other medical situation is it so hard to design an optimal pattern for treating patients in their homes, at clinics, and in hospitals. And in no other medical situation do the experts continue to differ so much among themselves about the preferred methods of prevention.

Dramatic gains have taken place in controlling tuberculosis but many problems of prevention and treatment remain. The initial optimistic forecast that the disease would soon be exterminated from the life of affluent nations has diminished.

Our options in seeking to bring the disease under effective control depend on our understanding of the strategic factors that help to spread it as well as of how best to influence the behavior of those afflicted by or exposed to it.

What then is the extent of our understanding?[1]

No one questions that the incidence of tuberculosis is closely correlated with socioeconomic determinants. But there is apparently no hard evidence that the rate of breakdown is closely correlated with poverty and economic distress. This is an important distinction. Active tuberculosis is more prevalent among the poor, but this does not imply that low economic status will result in a large number of breakdowns among people who are infected with the bacillus. There is no evidence to this effect.

While the number of new cases of tuberculosis has been declining in New York City over the past decades, there is no sound statistical information that would permit us to generalize about how fast tuberculosis is declining or whether the decline has begun to level off. There are no data that would enable us to differentiate among older persons who had been earlier infected who break down, younger persons whose tuberculosis becomes active, and older and younger people who have been infected who may, or may not, break down in the future. The presumptive evidence is that declines occurred in each of these populations but our knowledge is more impressionistic than statistical. We do know that many persons who today are being treated for active tuberculosis were treated at an earlier time but were not cured.

Another point and a crucial one with regard to effective planning and programing is that many who have active tuberculosis also suffer from other disabilities, such as old age, social marginality, alcoholism, and drug addiction.

Tuberculosis can appear as a singular or unique condition, but this is usually the exception.

Even though the number of new cases appears to be declining steadily, some new cases of moderately or even seriously advanced tuberculosis are reported. It is not true that a person with the disease can become seriously ill only after a long period of time. Tuberculosis is a disease with many variants, and some people get very sick very quickly. This being so, it is essential that hospital beds be available for such patients since definitive treatment for many moderately and, particularly, advanced cases cannot be instituted on an ambulatory basis.

A high proportion of new cases come to the attention of the medical authorities indirectly. Often a person who is admitted to a hospital for another condition is discovered to have tuberculosis by routine x-ray examination.

Much has been made in the past—and is still being made —of case finding. All sorts of alternative programs have adherents. However, the numbers identified through any of the established methods represent a small percentage of the total population that is screened. The question therefore must be raised whether it might not be preferable from the point of health needs of the community as a whole to add the resources so expended to the pool which is used to broaden and deepen the access particularly of the poor to general health services.

Among the poor—Negroes, Puerto Ricans, immigrants, the uneducated—"tuberculosis" is still a fearful term that carries ominous psychological as well as physical threats. People who learn that they have tuberculosis have every reason to be disturbed. A mother fears separation from her children and spouse, the man fears for his job, the drifter does not want to be separated from his cronies.

We know that even educated people in middle- and upper-income brackets frequently attempt to avoid learning what is wrong with them and when they find out they frequently refuse to follow the regimen prescribed by their physician. How much more likely this is to occur among the poor who have objective reasons to fear the additional burdens with which tuberculosis confronts them.

Another important consideration in programing for tuberculosis relates to the balance between inpatient and outpatient treatment facilities. Neither one nor the other can be relied upon exclusively. But the proper balance is not easy to find. How long should a patient be in a hospital? In part the answer is determined by his response to intensive therapy. How long will it take before his clinical symptoms are negative and how much longer before they are stabilized? The decision to release a patient also hinges in part on his home situation and on the probabilities of his cooperating as an outpatient. These are not easy judgments to make.

This last point suggests another. In the provision of medical care in general and in the treatment of tuberculosis in particular, too little attention has been paid to eliciting the full cooperation of the patient both in diagnosis and in therapy. The assumption that medical care is a service provided by a specialist to a layman is an error. There can be no proper health care without specialists, but there can be no effective health care without the involvement of the patient. The critical question is how to link more effectively patient and physician, patient and nurse, patient and hospital, patient and clinic.

There are specialists in tuberculosis who keep repeating that they "know how to cure tuberculosis." But do they really? The proponents of this doctrine imply that if they could go out into the community, find all the people with active tuberculosis, hold them prisoners for two years, and force them to take their medication, they could be discharged as cured. However in the course of this method of therapy many patients might lose their sanity or commit suicide. Only if we introduce a false dichotomy between the purely medical and the other aspects of a person's life can we talk about our ability to wipe out tuberculosis. Since, however, we can never distinguish so sharply between the purely medical and the purely social aspects of life, we must acknowledge that we do not know how to cure tuberculosis. That is the nub of the problem.

What then should be the new directions for action? Reference was made earlier to the economics of case finding. Let us look a little more closely at that problem. New York City is characterized by a continual stream of people into the city and an even greater movement of people within the city and out. Within ten months some public schools have more than a 100 percent turnover of their pupils. It is particularly difficult to do effective case finding under conditions of such high mobility. For the same reason it is not clear that efforts at tracking down contacts will necessarily pay off.

Clearly there is much to be said for tracking down contacts in a stable family in a stable neighborhood. If one of the family is identified as having active tuberculosis it would be well to institute prophylaxis with the others. But in New York City tuberculosis runs particularly high among single men who have no permanent domicile.

Moreover many persons who seek medical attention help to identify themselves. The problem of tuberculosis control in New York City may be no more than a footnote to the broader problem of providing health services for poor people. Without a basic minimum level of hospital and clinic services available to the poor, it may not prove possible to reach the many who have tuberculosis. There may be an analogy to malaria control in developing countries. After a certain point, no further progress can be made unless a certain minimum level of medical services becomes available to the general population.

Tuberculosis control must be integrated into a larger system of medical care. Admittedly, the patient with tuberculosis needs specialized treatment. But in the year 1969, in metropolitan centers, and particularly in ghettos, efforts to improve health through categorical programs in the absence of a minimum system of general medical services are neither sensible nor feasible.

Several reasons can be advanced in elaboration of this position. We noted earlier that many persons with tuberculosis are identified as a result of their being admitted to a hospital for other conditions but where a routine chest x-ray reveals that they have the disease. Clearly if the population at high risk had access to more medical care services, particularly within their own neighborhoods or close by,

a large number of active cases would be identified simply
as a by-product of the process whereby a resident sought
relief for a hacking cough or a mother brought her child
to the clinic because of a suspicious loss of weight and
energy.

The obverse should also be stressed. If people have relatively little access to health services, if they are not aware
of the symptoms of disease and of the ways that they can
be helped to alleviate and cure their conditions, they will
not respond adequately to a categorical program aimed at
the control of tuberculosis. How people react to any particular health program is closely linked to their attitudes
and experience with health services in general.

A related question is how to treat those who have been
identified as having active tuberculosis. This is the single
most difficult aspect of the problem. Finding the person
with the disease is important; even more important is to
determine an effective way of treating him. Despite the
revolution in chemotherapy the structure of providing care
for patients with tuberculosis has not been adequately
modified. With regard to the large number of marginal
persons, poorly educated, socially disorganized, who suffer
from tuberculosis, it is not possible to prescribe a therapeutic regimen based on their taking frequent drugs by
mouth, especially drugs that upset the system. But equivalent medication could be given by periodic injection and
a system could be established which would command the
requisite manpower to give the injections and provide incentives for the patients to cooperate in taking them. Then,

and only then, would the advances in therapeutics be effective for this difficult patient group.

Physicians have always assumed that medical care is a professional service to be rendered by an expert to a layman. Clearly there is much truth to this model when it comes to advanced therapeutics such as an operation or a series of x-ray treatments. But there is another model that provides a much closer fit when it comes to the diagnosis and treatment of many conditions, including tuberculosis. The physician may still have a critical role to play in one or another stage of the process of providing health care. But closer inspection reveals that the key to the process is not the physician–patient relation but rather the complex social and environmental conditions and circumstances that largely determine whether those who are ill will be identified; whether they will seek treatment; and most importantly whether they will follow the preferred regimen that will relieve them of their symptoms and condition. Since tuberculosis is a disease that can be treated effectively only over a period of many months, the social factors that will help to determine whether patients seek treatment and whether they follow the treatment that is prescribed will be of major importance in determining the success of any preventative, therapeutic, and rehabilitative program.

Three distinctions can be made among tuberculosis patients. One group consists of cooperative patients. The cooperative patient who has a cooperative family is relatively easy to discover and to treat. However, even for this patient, adjustments must be made. More clinics should be open in the evening and on weekends. It might even be desirable to locate a few clinics in areas of concentrated employment so that patients could be treated while continuing at work.

A second and more difficult group of patients are those who are willing to cooperate but who confront reality problems, such as the need for different housing arrangements to cut down the risks of contagion, and those who must change from full-time to part-time work as a result of the disease.

By definition the patients who confront the most serious reality problems are those who are poor and near-poor. Alone they cannot find larger apartments; if they stop working full time they need income supplement. They require not only medical attention but also assistance from the Housing Department, the Welfare Department, and other agencies of government. But it is difficult to work out a total program for a patient and his family and it is likely that before a program can be instituted he will fall through the cracks of the system and slip out of the hands of the physician.

The third subgroup is the most difficult of all; it is comprised of "marginal" people. This is a descriptive, not an invidious, term. These are persons with multiple problems, among which alcoholism and drug addiction are two of the important ones. Such people live on the fringe of society. They are a constant source of infection and breakdown. They infect not only each other but others as well.

We are still groping to design an effective plan to deal with socially disorganized persons who have tuberculosis.

What then should a large city aim to do? We need periodic testing of the population to determine the trends in the incidence and prevalence of tuberculosis. We need periodic bench marks to assess changes and developments in the situation.

Second, we need better health services for the ghetto population so situated that they will be encouraged to use them. We must rely increasingly on self-referrals to identify persons with tuberculosis.

Third, it is essential to involve the ghetto population directly in both case-finding and therapeutics.

A specialist in chest diseases should be on the front line of a therapeutic program once the diagnosis has been made so that the disease can be brought under preliminary control. If the patient cannot be relied upon to take his medicine by mouth, an indigenous worker must be found who will be willing to climb three flights of stairs twice a week to give him his injection. To teach an indigenous worker to do this job might take a few hours of training, surely not more than a few days. Many people in the ghetto would welcome the opportunity to become a member of a health team and to have a job which is socially useful.

It will be more difficult to bring about the improved coordination between hospital and clinic which is urgently required if full advantage is to be taken of the modern treatment of tuberculosis, and it will be even more difficult to secure the cooperation among the several departments of city government which is required if medical care is to be provided within a supportive social environment.

Finally, the voluntary organizations which have played so prominent a part in the program up to now must recognize that we do not have adequate answers for the effective control and eradication of tuberculosis in our large metropolitan centers and that it is their responsibility and their opportunity to foster experimental programs aimed at finding these answers. We have come a long way but we still have a long way to go. The last steps may prove to be the most difficult.

◦ 19 ◦
Perspectives: A Forward View

This book has presented a commentary on the changing structure of health services in the United States during the past quarter century with particular emphasis on the rapid changes that followed the introduction of Medicare in 1965. Unlike the statements of many both within and outside the health professions who have a clear sense of the direction which "the system" should take to guarantee all citizens the benefits of modern medicine, the present effort is primarily analytical and evaluative rather than exhortatory. It has sought to delineate the ways in which American medicine is rooted in the larger fabric of our national life and to indicate the changes that must be made in our values and institutions before the health industry can be significantly restructured. Those who have read this far know that the author is not opposed to restructuring but that he believes that the serious student must weigh proposals with regard to both feasibility and potential results, not only for improvements in medical care but for the other goals and values we hope to protect and enhance.

Continuity characterizes the life of a nation except dur-

ing a major revolution. Therefore it may be useful to look
back briefly before looking ahead in the hope of uncover-
ing some of the major linkages between changes in medicine and changes in the broader environment which may
cast a shadow of likely changes in the future.

Since the beginning of World War II, the economic
foundations of modern medicine have been transformed.
In absolute and relative terms both the consumer and government spend much more on health services. Health has
become one of the nation's most important industries, and
the hospital is its site. Nonprofit and commercial insurance
play a major role in the financing of hospital care. For the
first time the wages and salaries of health workers approximate the earnings of workers with comparable education
and skill in other sectors of the economy. From these and
other changes we conclude that a rapidly expanding, high-
income economy has sufficient flexibility built into it to
find the large additional sums—and to design new mechanisms for raising them—to supply the consuming public
with more and better services.

In light of the major adaptations that have occurred in
the economics of the health services industry during the
last quarter century, we question whether putative per
diem hospital costs of even $200 would require a major
overhaul of the present system. Such an increase would be
of the same order of magnitude as the ones to which the
system has adapted in the recent past.

We cannot view with equanimity the continued and
steep rise in medical and hospital costs. On the other hand
it should not be taken as evidence of the imminent collapse

of the present system. Dr. John Knowles, in a recent in-
terview reported in *Medical Economics*, contemplated per
diem costs rising to $300, $400, and $500 without conclud-
ing that such costs would require that American medical
care be completely restructured.

A look backward suggests that the potential trends in
national and family income, juxtaposed with potential
costs of health care, will not create a disequilibrium which
would make it impossible for the present structure to continue to operate. There are many Cassandras, and they may
turn out to be right, but a reassessment of the recent past
does not add to their credibility.

With regard to manpower, there has been a slow but
steady increase in the number of medical schools, enrollment, and graduates during the last decades. We have
added to our physician pool by licensing large numbers
of foreign-trained physicians who have come to the United
States for graduate study or to live. Leaving aside such important questions as whether the rich United States should
draw physicians from less affluent countries and whether
all foreign-trained physicians meet our minimum standards, the prospect is that our domestic training capacity
will expand and our net gains from immigration will continue; we will maintain approximately the ratio of physicians to population which has been maintained since
World War II. Many Americans do not see a physician as
often as their conditions would indicate or as they would
desire, but the outlook for the near future will not worsen.

The ability of the health services industry to broaden
and deepen the services it provides the American people

reflects in large measure the large and continuing expansion in allied health manpower to a point where today 9 out of 10 workers in the industry are persons other than physicians. While there have been and continue to be bottlenecks in many parts of this complex manpower structure, which has over 40 professional branches and many more on the para-professional level, ever larger numbers of trained personnel are attracted to the industry. There is every reason to believe that the additional personnel that will be required in the years ahead can be attracted, trained, and retained. In fact, this task should prove less difficult now that various levels of government have taken a more active role in financing the education and training of health workers and since their salaries and wages have become more nearly competitive with those in other industries.

In short, while there is little prospect that all manpower shortages will disappear in the near future—they may not even ease—there is no basis for believing that they will worsen. On balance, the odds favor a closer match between demand and supply in the years ahead.

A third arena of concern can be subsumed under the rubric of "the delivery of medical services." Let us see what has happened in the recent past. The hospital has an ever more important role in the delivery of medical services, although regrettably it has concentrated almost exclusively on inpatients. There has been a growth of various types of group practice; but for the most part these have not been part of a comprehensive system to meet all health needs. In the last few years, largely under the impetus of the Office of Economic Opportunity, an effort has been made to establish comprehensive health clinics in ghetto areas and in a limited number of centers of rural poverty in the hope of bringing essential health services closer to the resident population and at the same time involving them in designing the type of services they require and providing opportunity for the indigenous population to be part of the team providing these services.

Some modest efforts have also been made to bring more regional planning into the health services industry in the expectation that both duplications and deficiencies could be eliminated. At best progress along these lines has been modest. Health services continue to be subject to planning and control—only at the margins. Similarly, there has been some evidence of desire among management, labor, and consumer groups to become part of the decision-making mechanisms. Since these groups put up most of the money, they want to have more of a say. The day when physicians, hospital administrators, and Blue Cross officials were able to decide on a course of action among themselves appears to be almost over.

What does this sketch tell us about the likely shape of things to come? It suggests that while changes in the delivery system have occurred, these changes have been modest. There has been a steady drift toward more full-time physicians on the staff of major teaching hospitals. In many communities the hospital's X-ray and laboratory and other facilities are used by the attending staff to provide services for their private ambulatory patients. In large cities, the poor and near-poor have pressed the hospitals

to establish, expand, and improve emergency room services. But these developments indicate that the basic pattern
for the delivery of health services has been changing slowly.
The private practitioner, alone or in group practice, continues to dominate the scene.

While recent trends have started to disturb the doctor,
particularly the schism between the full-time hospital staff
and himself, his services have been and continue to be in
high demand. Consequently he is not likely to take the
lead to change the status quo. He has plenty of patients
and earns a good income.

The outlook then is for only modest changes in the delivery system in the years ahead. The university and the
large teaching hospital with full-time staff will probably
become dominant. While the British are attempting to
build bridges between their GP's and their specialists who
are hospital-based, the split in this country between those
in private and full-time hospital practice is likely to widen.
If the law is altered—as it may well be—to permit physicians to incorporate and to offer more leverage for hospitals
and other corporate structures to organize medical resources and to provide medical services, the rate of transformation may be speeded up considerably. The medical
services industry would then be on the way to shifting from
one characterized by private practitioners to corporate
entities.

An associated trend will probably be the increase of salaried physicians on government payrolls and in nonprofit
organizations supported by government funds. This would
permit the delivery of more and better services to hitherto

neglected population groups such as the urban and rural poor. Since the expansion of quality services to the poor cannot possibly be made by replicating the system now in use for providing services to the middle class, the only prospect of success would be through a radical revision of the delivery system involving hospital-based full-time staff working with a broad allied health team which would include indigenous members from the population to be served. If government allocations make it possible for young physicians to earn a good livelihood and if the co-operating institutions were provided sufficient latitude to innovate, the prospects for constructive change might be favorably assessed. The primary reason is that many young men now in medical school and those who are likely to enter in the future belong to a new generation. They want to make a good living, but they also have other values, including a more meaningful relationship to their society.

While the delivery of health services has been changed relatively little in the recent past, there is a fair chance that it will undergo accelerated changes in the future in response to the growing dominance of the teaching hospital with full-time staff and the erosion of the solo practitioner. Changes will accelerate as medical services are increasingly organized and delivered by corporate enterprises, and as a significant number of young physicians become interested in social medicine, in an effort to improve health services for the poor.

As we have seen, the American people have tended to equate health with improved medical care. They have paid relatively little attention to such matters as population in-

creases, income, accident prevention, alcohol, drugs, cigarettes, education, and employment policies in health preservation and rehabilitation. Yet the evidence grows daily that
significant gains in longevity, the reduction of morbidity,
and improvement in the quality of life may be more closely
linked to these ancillary developments than to an increase
in medical services per se. We have only recently begun
to appreciate the importance of liberalizing our laws and
practices with respect to birth control and abortion. Clearly
much human misery can be avoided if children are born
only to parents who want them and are able to care for
them. It is likely that we will see substantial gains along
this frontier. The challenge of genetic counseling and intervention lies in the more distant future.

We have only recently become aware that in the rich
United States many adults and children do not eat enough
or do not eat the right foods. Part of these dietary deficiencies are a direct consequence of lack of income. While
additional research is required to trace the disabilities that
grow out of malnutrition and hunger, we know that in
this area corrective action is long overdue. Now that the
issue has been precipitated in Congress and among the
public it is likely that corrective actions will be speeded.

The slaughter on the roads continues apace. However,
stories in the press and the threats of damage suits have
led the automotive companies to exercise greater caution
in design and to call back defective units. But in light of
the amount of premature death and serious disability
caused by highway accidents, we are still doing too little
on this front. It is difficult to foresee whether the public

will press for major reforms. It appears to be questionable.

We have become alerted in recent years to the ravages of various addictive agents—alcohol, drugs, and tobacco. The per capita consumption of alcohol continues to rise. The use of drugs is steadily increasing and their sale is being pushed among children in junior and senior high school. Our enforcement policies are weak and our rehabilitation efforts continue inadequate. Here is an important health problem which is largely out of control.

With respect to the use of tobacco, the trend is somewhat equivocal. During the last years, there has been considerable effort on the part of both the federal government and voluntary health agencies to launch and carry out a sizable campaign about the dangers of smoking. This campaign has had some effect. But the tobacco industry has attempted to attract new consumers while holding on to those who now smoke. To date the public does not appear willing to consider a more radical program aimed at restricting tobacco advertising or to take other actions, such as punitive taxes, to reduce the sale of cigarettes.

While health education has been a recognized field of public health for many years and while the communications industry, particularly the monthly magazines, bring health information to their readers, there is a large gap between what people need to know for the protection of their health and the information they have. Moreover, health education goes beyond providing simple information and includes the challenge of getting people to act in accordance with the knowledge they have. In light of the many years young people remain in school and the penetration of radio and television, the potential for improved health information can be better exploited. Since the individual must initiate the process of seeking health services, his failure to understand, to act, or to act wisely can make a mockery of attempts to improve other segments of the health system.

During the past decades we have come to recognize that there are close links between the psyche and the soma and that a man disturbed in his spirit is not likely to feel or be well. Moreover we have noted the important links between a person's health and his ability to function productively as a member of his community. Despite this understanding we have done relatively little to assure that all persons able and willing to work have the opportunity to do so. While we have expanded federal and state programs of vocational rehabilitation and introduced many new employment programs, we have fallen far short of providing a job for everybody who needs and desires one. Here is another sphere where we can add considerably to the health and well-being of large numbers of poor and otherwise handicapped people by taking every feasible action to achieve a full employment economy.

We must not continue to ignore or minimize the potential gains from approaching the challenge of better health not only frontally, by expanding and improving our system of medical care, but also by a flank approach through improved policies and programs in such critically important areas as income, education, and employment. Of all the lessons we can extract from the recent past, the most basic is to understand the potentialities of contributing to better health through improving the environment.

This exercise in probing the determinants of our health system may leave many readers dissatisfied. We have been unable to discern even the shadowy outlines of a panacea for all the ills that are imbedded in our present structure and operations. Moreover, we have been unable to conclude that, even with the passage of additional time, most of the serious defects are likely to be eradicated. Such an eventuality does not appear likely.

But we can hope that a better educated and more affluent people will insure that the existing system is modified to accomplish three major objectives: that the advances in science and technology will be exploited so that our health will be better protected and maintained; that the resources of men and money devoted to this end will be effectively utilized; that those without adequate income are not arbitrarily barred from the benefits that the system is able to provide.

Progress towards these three objectives will not be made quickly or easily. And as progress is made, however slowly, new problems will be precipitated and new potentialities opened up. The next generation, like the last, will confront the same issue—how best to improve an imperfect system of health care within a democratic structure which itself is and must inevitably remain imperfect even while it is being improved.

❧ Notes ❧

1. Perspectives: A Retrospective View

1. U.S. Dept. of Commerce, Bureau of the Census, *Statistical Abstract of the United States: 1968* (Washington D.C., 1968), p. 63.

2. George Ball, Keynote Address, in U.S. Dept. of Health, Education, and Welfare, *Summary: The Secretary's Regional Conference on Health Care Costs, New York City, January, 1969* (Washington, D.C., 1969).

3. Eli Ginzberg, "Army Hospitalization: Retrospect and Prospect," *Bulletin of the United States Army Medical Department,* 8 (January, 1948), 38 ff.

4. Eli Ginzberg, *A Pattern for Hospital Care* (New York, Columbia University Press, 1949).

5. Eli Ginzberg, "What Every Economist Should Know About Health and Medicine," *American Economic Review,* 44 (March, 1954), 104 ff.

6. Eli Ginzberg, Papers and Proceedings of Symposium on "Economics of Medical Care," *American Economic Review,* 41, (May, 1951), 624.

7. *Ibid.,* pp. 621 and 623.

8. Eli Ginzberg, "Communications," *American Economic Review,* 44 (December, 1954), 928 ff.

9. Eli Ginzberg, Chairman of the Committee on the Function of Nursing, *A Program for the Nursing Profession* (New York, Macmillan, 1948).

10. National Manpower Council, *A Policy for Scientific and*

Professional Manpower (New York, Columbia University Press, 1953), p. 240.

11. Ginzberg, "What Every Economist Should Know," p. 115.

12. Eli Ginzberg, "The Ills That Beset the British Health Plan," *The Modern Hospital*, 74 (May, 1950), 138.

13. Ginzberg, "Communications," p. 931.

14. Ginzberg, "What Every Economist Should Know," p. 118.

15. Ginzberg, Papers and Proceedings, p. 624.

16. *Journal of the Mount Sinai Hospital of New York*, 19 (March-April, 1953), 734 ff.

17. Eli Ginzberg et al., *The Ineffective Soldier: Lessons for Management and the Nation*, 3 vols. (New York, Columbia University Press, 1959): *Journal of the Mount Sinai Hospital*, p. 736.

18. Eli Ginzberg and Peter Rogatz, M.D., *Planning for Better Hospital Care* (New York, Kings Crown Press, 1961).

19. Harry I. Greenfield with Carol Brown, *Allied Health Manpower: Trends and Prospects* (New York, Columbia University Press, 1969).

20. See also Eli Ginzberg, "The Hospital and the Community: Some Dynamic Interrelations," in *The Impact of Antibiotics on Medicine and Society*, Iago Galdston, ed. (New York, International Universities Press, 1958), pp. 187 ff.; and Ginzberg, "The Political Economy of Health," *Bulletin of the New York Academy of Medicine*, 41 (October, 1965), 1015 ff.

2. *Facts and Fancies About Medical Care*

A shortened version of this chapter appeared in *The American Journal of Public Health*, Vol. 59, No. 5 (May, 1969).

1. Sir Geoffrey Vickers, "What Sets the Goals of Public Health?" *Lancet,* 1 (March 22, 1958), 599-604.

2. Metropolitan Life Insurance Co., *Statistical Bulletin* (May, 1967), pp. 2-6; David Rutstein, *The Coming Revolution in Medicine* (Cambridge, M.I.T. Press, 1967), pp. 13-15; and U.S. Dept. of Health, Education, and Welfare, National Center for Health Statistics, Series 3, No. 1, *The Change in Mortality Trend in the United States* (Washington D.C., 1964), pp. 40-41.

3. The Health Services Industry

This chapter is adapted from U.S. Depts. of Labor–Health, Education, and Welfare, "Training Health Service Workers: The Critical Challenge," *Proceedings of the Conference on Job Development and Training for Workers in Health Services, February 14-17, 1966* (Washington D.C., 1966), pp. 16 ff.

1. Donald Yett, "The Nursing Shortage and the Nurse Training Act of 1964," *Industrial and Labor Relations Review,* 19 (January, 1966), 190-200.

4. Hospitals and Collective Bargaining

This essay is adapted from a chapter in a forthcoming volume on *Emerging Sectors of Collective Bargaining* to be published under the auspices of the Temple University School of Business Administration.

1. U.S. Dept. of Health, Education, and Welfare, Public Health Service Publication No. 1509, *Health Resources Statistics: 1968* (Washington D.C., 1968), p. 223, Table 149.

5. *What Price Medicaid?*

Reprinted with minor changes by permission of the Reporter Magazine Company from *The Reporter*, January 25, 1968.

1. Title XIX Fact Sheets and U.S. Dept. of Health, Education, and Welfare, Social and Rehabilitation Service, Assistance Payments Administration, Division of Program Operations, "Status of Medical Assistance Programs under Title XIX as of December 1, 1967."

2. Computed from statistics furnished in N.Y. State Dept. of Social Services, *Medicaid: Year in Review, March, 1966-April, 1967* (Albany, July, 1967) and supplementary services and expenditure data.

3. *Medical Tribune,* December 7, 1967.

4. *Medical Tribune,* November 30, 1967.

6. *The Physician and Market Power*

Adapted from U.S. Dept. of Health, Education, and Welfare, "Manpower and Market Power," *Report of the National Conference on Medical Costs* (Washington D.C., June, 1967).

1. B. E. Balfe and M. E. McNamara, *Survey of Medical Groups in the U.S., 1965* (New York, American Medical Association, 1968), pp. 11, 40-49, and 77-88; and M. Terris, "Origins and Growth of Group Practice," *Bulletin of the New York Academy of Medicine* (November, 1968), pp. 1229-81.

2. New York *Times,* December 12, 1967.

3. Carnegie Corporation–Commonwealth Fund Conference, *The Crisis in Medical Education,* (Fort Lauderdale, Fla., February, 1966).

7. *The Physician Shortage Reconsidered*

Reprinted with minor changes by permission of the *New England Journal of Medicine*, 275 (July 14, 1966), 85-87.

1. U.S. Dept. of Health, Education, and Welfare, *The Advancement of Medical Research and Education,* Final Report of the Secretary's Consultants on Medical Research and Education (Washington D.C., 1958); HEW, Public Health Service Bulletin No. 709, *Physicians for a Growing America,* Report of the Surgeon General's Consultant Group on Medical Education (Washington D.C., 1959); HEW, Public Health Service Bulletin No. 1001, *Manpower for Medical Research: Requirements and Resources, 1965-1970,* Report No. 3 of Consultant Group on Medical Research (Washington D.C., 1963); *A National Program to Conquer Heart Disease, Cancer, and Stroke,* Report of the President's Commission on Heart Disease, Cancer, and Stroke (Washington D.C., 1965); and *Report of the National Advisory Commission on Health Manpower* (Washington D.C., 1967), Vol. I.

2. Carnegie Corporation—Commonwealth Fund Conference, *The Crisis in Medical Education* (Fort Lauderdale, Fla., February, 1966).

3. The Census reported a decline of population growth rate in 1968 to 1 percent of total population, lowest figure since 1940.

4. Rashi Fein, *The Doctor Shortage* (Washington D.C., Brookings Institution, 1967), pp. 140-43.

5. A. B. Bergman, S. W. Dassel, and R. J. Wedgwood, "Time-Motion Study of Practicing Pediatricians," *Pediatrics,* 38 (August, 1966), 254-63.

8. *The Medical Specialist: The Obstetrician*

Based on an address given at the annual staff dinner, Department of Obstetrics and Gynecology, Downstate Medical Center, New York, October 11, 1967.

1. E. M. Craft, "Consumer Income and Expenditures for Health Care," *Journal of the American Medical Association,* 207 (January 6, 1969), 139-40,

2. C. N. Theodore and E. A. Jokiel, *Distribution of Physicians, Hospitals, and Hospital Beds in the United States, 1966* (New York, American Medical Association, 1967), pp. 122-41.

3. American Medical Association, Council on Medical Education, *Medical Education in the United States, 1967-1968* (New York, 1968), pp. 2027-35.

4. *The Training and Responsibilities of the Midwife* (New York, Josiah Macy Jr. Foundation, 1967), pp. x and 149-55.

5. U.S. Dept. of Health, Education, and Welfare, Public Health Service Publication No. 1509, *Health Resources Statistics: 1968* (Washington DC., 1968), pp. 133-34.

9. *New Missions for Public Health*

Reported with minor changes by permission of the American Public Health Association from "A Manpower Strategy for Public Health," *American Journal of Public Health,* 57 (April, 1967), 588 ff.

10. *The Woman Physician*

Based on U.S. Dept. of Labor, Women's Bureau, "Professional Manpower for an Affluent Society," report on a conference, *The Fuller Utilization of the Woman Physician* (Washington D.C., July, 1968), pp. 3-8.

1. Estimated from U.S. Dept. of Labor, Women's Bureau, "Facts on Prospective and Practicing Women in Medicine" (Washington D.C., 1968); American Medical Association, Council on Medical Education, *Medical Education in the United States, 1967-1968* (New York, 1968), p. 2085.

2. U.S. Dept. of Labor, Wage and Labor Standards Administration, *Background Facts of Women Workers in the United States* (Washington D.C., September, 1968), p. 9, Table 6; and Labor Dept., "Fact Sheet of Trends in Educational Attainment of Women," WB 68-154 (Washington D.C., April, 1968).

3. Labor Dept., *Background Facts of Women Workers*, p. 15, Table 12.

4. National Academy of Sciences, *Doctorate Recipients from United States Universities*, Publication No. 1489 (Washington D.C., 1967), ch. 5.

5. Carol Lopate, *Women in Medicine* (Baltimore, Johns Hopkins University Press, 1968).

6. AMA, *Medical Education in the United States*, p. 2013, Table 14.

11. *The Expanding Supply*

Reprinted from Foreword to *Allied Health Manpower: Trends and Prospects* by Harry I. Greenfield with Carol A. Brown (New York, Columbia University Press, 1969).

1. This is the number of employees on payrolls in the civilian health service industry. Another million persons are employed in the military services, in industries related to health services (namely, drug manufacture and trade), and in health occupations outside the health services industry (namely, vet-

erinary medicine). U.S. Dept. of Health, Education, and Welfare, Public Health Service, *Health Manpower Source Book,* Section 18 (Washington D.C., 1964).

2. Assistant-physician training program, directed by Dr. Eugene Stead, Duke University (cf. "More than a Nurse, Less than a Doctor," *Look,* September 6, 1966, pp. 58-61); experimental program at Health Sciences Center, Temple University.

12. *Nursing Realities*

Adapted with permission of the American Journal of Nursing Company from "Nursing and Manpower Realities," *Nursing Outlook* (November, 1967), 26-29.

1. U.S. Dept. of Health, Education, and Welfare, Public Health Service Publication No 992, *Toward Quality in Nursing: Needs and Goals,* Report of the Surgeon General's Consultant Group on Nursing (Washington D.C., 1963).

2. American Nurses Association, *Facts About Nursing* (New York, 1968), p 7.

3. *Ibid.,* p. 107, Table 4.

4. *Ibid.,* p. 90, chart 6.

5. Eli Ginzberg, Chairman of the Committee on the Function of Nursing, *A Program for the Nursing Profession* (New York, Macmillan, 1948).

6. ANA, *Facts About Nursing,* pp. 104-12.

13. *Clinical Laboratory Personnel*

Completely rewritten from "The Social and Economic Outlook," *American Journal of Medical Technology,* 34 (March, 1968).

1. Most of the data for this chapter are from National Committee for Careers in Medical Technology, *Background Material for National Conference, October 11-13, 1967* (College Park, University of Maryland, 1967).

14. *Social Workers*

Adapted from "Manpower Planning for Social Work," *Use of Personnel in Child Welfare Agencies,* Helen Fradkin, ed. (New York, Columbia University School of Social Work, Arden House Conference, October 20-November 3, 1966), pp. 1 ff.

1. U.S. Dept. of Health, Education, and Welfare, *Closing the Gap in Social Work Manpower,* Report of the Departmental Task Force on Social Work Education and Manpower (Washington, D.C., 1965). The discussion here of programmatic recommendations for the enhancement of manpower in the field of professional social work is based upon the concluding chapter, which summarizes the Task Force findings and proposals.

15. *The Mentally Handicapped*

Reprinted with substantial changes by permission of the Johns Hopkins Press from "The Mentally Handicapped in a Technological Society," in *The Biosocial Basis of Mental Retardation,* Sonia F. Osler and Robert E. Cooke, eds. (Baltimore, Johns Hopkins Press, 1965).

1. U.S. Dept. of Labor, Task Force on Manpower Conservation, *One-Third of a Nation: A Report of Young Men Found Unqualified for Military Service* (Washington D.C., 1964).

2. Eli Ginzberg and Douglas Bray, *The Uneducated* (New York, Columbia University Press, 1953); and Ginzberg et al.,

The Ineffective Soldier: Lessons for Management and the Nation, 3 vols. (New York, Columbia University Press, 1959).

16. *Priorities for Psychiatry*

Reprinted with substantial changes by permission of the Council of State Governments and the Northeast State Governments Conference on Mental Health from "Manpower and Mental Health," *Summary of Proceedings, Northeast State Governments Conference on Mental Health, September 12-14, 1966* (Chicago, Interstate Clearing House on Mental Health, 1966), pp. 2ff.

17. *Mental Health in Industry*

Reprinted with changes by permission of the Industrial Medical Association from "Technological Change and Adjustment to Work," *Journal of Occupational Medicine,* 9 (May, 1967), 232 ff.

1. Eli Ginzberg, James K. Anderson, and John L. Herma, *The Optimistic Tradition and American Youth* (New York, Columbia University Press, 1962).

18. *Tuberculosis Control*

Adapted from a presentation at the Spring Conference of the New York Tuberculosis and Health Association, April 23, 1968.

1. New York State, Council of the TB and Health Associations, *A Modern Attack on an Urban Health Problem,* Report of the Task Force on Tuberculosis in New York City (Albany, 1968).

Index

4